GET UP & GO

A GUIDE FOR THE
MATURE TRAVELER

GET UP & GO

GENE & ADELE
MALOTT

GATEWAY BOOKS

Printed in the United States of America

Gateway Books
San Francisco

12 11 10 9 8 7 6 5 4 3 2 1

ACKNOWLEDGEMENTS

Our thanks to these people and organizations, whose help enabled us to make the intricacies of travel easier to understand:

Dawn Ringel, Institute of Certified Travel Agents; Ray M. Greenly, American Society of Travel Agents; Shirley Norton, Bank of America; Jerri Eskow, Deak International; Stephen Forsyth, Forsyth Travel Library; M.A. Uffer, International Association for Medical Assistance to Travellers (IAMAT); Denise Madden and Dr. Arthur H. Kibbe, American Pharmaceutical Association. Ray Todd, Kampgrounds of America; Carolyn Speidel, Cruise Lines International Association; Kathy Lane, The Weather Channel; Michele Kelley, American Hotel & Motel Association; Jerry Cheske, American Automobile Association (AAA); Dr. James W. Kazura, chief of the Division of Geographic Medicine, Case Western Reserve University; Rosamond R. Dewart, Travelers' Health Section, Division of Quarantine, Centers for Disease Control; Frances Jones, Bureau of Consular Affairs, U.S. Department of State; Jackie Lang, Recreation Vehicle Industry Association; Terry Denny, International Air Transport Association; Patricia Duricka, National Railroad Passenger Corp. (Amtrak); Jackie Bellar, National Tour Association; David V. Lippincott, immediate past president, National Tour Association; Warren Lerude, author, *American Commander in Spain*; Patricia Sze, Berlitz Lanuage Centers.

And our special thanks to Jim Carney, whose eagle eye and sharp editor's pencil helped keep the grammatical demons at bay; and to Tamara Charland, whose research helped us to keep the facts straight.

— Gene & Adele Malott

Contents

I GETTING SET

II WAYS TO GO

III BEING THERE

IV PLACES

Dedicated
To the journey
. . . and to the friends and memories we make enroute.

I

GETTING SET

Seniors have more freedom to travel than anyone else.
Here's how to make the most of it.

CHAPTER 1

THE SAVVY SENIOR

| How to Become a Travel 'Insider' |

S eniors who travel can be divided into two kinds of people, a travel expert once told us: members and non-members. That's not quite accurate. There is a third kind: insiders. Insiders are those who take joy in the mechanics of travel as well as the places they travel to. Insiders, while they don't necessarily travel on the cheap, search for the best travel deals — read "values" — they can find. They take pleasure in learning ways to find them.

Insiders travel the way they want to, to places they want to, at the pace they want to. And they know how to check out the details.

Insiders rarely have a bad travel experience, for they do their homework and know how to make a trip work for them — even a trip that takes unexpected turns.

Though it may be your first major trip, you can still be an insider — an insider's bags needn't be plastered with travel stickers. Carrying around dozens of credit cards and club memberships doesn't make you an insider, either. Carrying around a lot of accumulated information, a guidebook with a map and a head full of good sense *can* make you an insider.

"INNER TRAVELING"

Being a travel insider is almost a state of mind. It requires a chain of thinking that moves from (a) I can have a good trip, to (b) I know how to have a good trip, to (c) I will have a good trip. Call it "inner traveling."

13

Inner Traveling, like Inner Golf, Inner Tennis or Inner Anything Else, starts with some imagination — some daydreaming.
Close your eyes, lean back and imagine yourself having the best
trip of your life — try to picture yourself exactly where you want
to be, doing exactly what you want to do. Then develop the
know-how to get out and do it.

This book assumes you (a) want to have a good trip. It
concentrates on (b) how you can have a good trip. And if you
take the advice to heart (c), you will have a good trip.

It will, in summary, tell you lots of those things you need to
know to become a travel insider.

You already started, in fact, when you began reading *Get Up
And Go!*; you did your first insider act.

WHAT'S A "SENIOR," ANYHOW?

The reader-board at the big motel in Winnemucca, Nev., said,
"Discounts for Those Over 65, and AARP Members." It raises the
question:

When do you become a senior traveler? At 65?

Not at all. You officially become a senior traveler whenever
you're smart enough to shell out $5 to join AARP, so you can get
$5.50 off a $55 room.

Well, you can do that at age 50.

You can become a card-carrying senior traveler at an even
younger age. Many travel deals for "those over 55" or other
specified age really mean that only one spouse has to be the
specified age. And many senior-citizen offers are for travelers as
young as 45. Once there was even a club that offered motel
discounts of up to 20 percent for those who'd just turned 40!

It bears out the message that when you hear talk about
"senior travel," it doesn't necessarily mean "travel for old
people." Rather, it means travel for those who've been around
long enough to have the common sense to look for the best deals.

DEALS FOR SENIORS

Travel deals are everywhere, for everybody.

Almost any traveler, young or old, who spends enough time
and knows where to look can take advantage of some kind of

special deal — 30-day-advance fares, "hidden-city" fares, auto-rental discounts, off-season rates, twofers and the like.

With the possible exception of meals, a traveler who pays full rate on anything is probably on an expense account. And even the cost of eating out in many cities can be reduced by purchase of a "Discount Dining Club" coupon book full of twofers, or by eating early.

As senior citizens, though, we are twice-blessed. Not only can we use the discounts that everybody else gets, but we get special discounts of our own.

Remember, you don't have to be retired to join AARP—just 50 or more. You do have to be mature — that is, 55 or older — to join Mature Outlook and take advantage of their deals.

You don't have to join anything to get bargains, though. A source that lists literally hundreds of senior travel deals is Caroline & Walter Weintz's book, *The Discount Guide for Travelers Over 55* (E.P. Dutton, New York), available for $8 or less at most large bookstores.

Many travel deals are moving targets — seasonal, subject to instant cancellation or the like. Many of those listed as examples in this book will be gone by the time you get around to using them. For that reason, you need to subscribe to an up-to-date travel newsletter (see Chapter 4 for some of the best ones). A good one is *The Mature Traveler* ($21.97 per year, P.O. Box 50820, Reno, NV 89513), the only subscription newsletter we know with current deals and special trips just for senior travelers. It's published by the authors of this book.

What kind of deals are offered to senior travelers? Here are some that were recently listed in *The Mature Traveler*. Be sure to write or phone on any of these before you make firm plans.

CRUISE DEALS

Premier Cruise Line offered this deal on its popular Bahamas cruise: For $595 — about 10 percent off — those over 60 get a four-night cruise, three nights' accommodations near Disney World in Orlando, Fla., free rental car and free admissions to Disney World and Epcot Center. Meals on the ship, of course, were included, though meals ashore were not. Whenever you can travel to any popular destination for less than $100 a day, you've got a real bargain. Other recent cruise deals included:

Florida-Bahama cruises on SeaEscape and Discovery cruises for seniors at 10 percent off regular prices — for as low as $79 a day.

Up to $800 savings for two — one had to be 65 or older — on autumn Chandris Fantasy Cruises from New York to the Caribbean. That's 25 percent off.

Up to $400 off — about 18 percent of the published cost — for those over 50 on a Taylor Tours 14-day trans-Panama cruise that also visited Curacao, Cartagena and the Mexican Riviera. That was a special positioning cruise — a one-time cruise that takes a ship from its old home port to a new one.

Your travel agent also could have alerted you to these senior specials.

DEALS ON TRAINS

Yes, the trains still run — especially in Europe. In the United States and in some European countries, seniors are entitled to deep discounts on train travel.

Amtrak gives 25 percent off all one-way coach fares once you turn 65. And all you have to do is ask the ticket agent.

The Canadian national railway, Via Rail, gives seniors 33 percent off — mature travelers can take the continent's longest rail trip, four days and 3,639 miles from Halifax to Vancouver, for only $228, a $113 saving. ☎ Phone toll-free 800/361-3663 for tickets and schedules.

Travelers over 59 get 15 percent discounts on BritRail first-class travel. Ask your travel agent.

France's Carte Vermeil provides railway discounts as well as cut-rate admissions to all museums. Write the French National Railroad office in New York City, or ask your travel agent.

For even cheaper travel, Greyhound has a 10 percent senior citizen discount nationwide.

DISCOUNT ADMISSIONS

Golden Age Passports are free lifetime passes to U.S. national parks, monuments and recreation areas, issued to those 62 and older. In addition, the passports give you 50 percent off the use fees for such things as boating, camping and parking. To get a Golden Age Passport, apply in person and show proof of age at any National Park Service office. Check your local phone book to find the location.

Thousands of attractions like these around the country also offer senior travelers discounts on admissions: the Queen Mary and Spruce Goose in Long Beach, Calif.; Cypress Gardens in Florida; Winterthur Museum in Delaware; San Francisco's Blue & Gold Fleet bay cruises; the Ashland (Oregon), Shakespeare Festival . . . the list is almost endless.

DEALS ON LODGINGS

Here are some typical deals for 49ers-plus at inns:

Atlas Hotels "Gold Club," for couples with one spouse over 55, offers discounts up to 20 percent in San Diego (Mission Valley Inn and others), the Southwest and Mexico. (Write 500 Hotel Circle N., San Diego, CA 92108; ☎ toll-free 800/854-2608; in California 800/542-6082.)

Hotel Bedford near San Francisco's Union Square offers anyone over 60 varying discounts that have ranged up to 25 percent, plus theater, dining and shopping packages. Loew's L'Enfant Plaza in Washington, D.C., gives seniors 60 and over 20 percent discounts on rooms and meals. Almost every hotel and motel in the United States and Canada, in fact, has a senior discount, some of them huge. Look at the biggest chains:

Marriott Hotels' Leisurelife program offers those over 62 discounts of 25 percent on dining, 50 percent on rooms and 10 percent on some items in hotel gift shops. (Write Marriott's Leisurelife Program, P.O. Box 10489, Rockville, MD 20850.)

Westin Hotels in Texas offer 50 percent off lodging and 10 percent off meals for anyone 60 and over.

There are also half-off deals for mature travelers at Hiltons and Omni Internationals, and lesser discounts at all the other chains. To get most of these discounts, all you have to do is ask.

Overseas, the Swiss Hotel Association puts out a brochure, *Season for Seniors*, listing hotels in that country providing discounts. Write Swiss National Tourist Office, 608 Fifth Avenue, New York, NY 10020.

AIRLINE DEALS

Airline deals for seniors change as fast as their fares — and that amounts to several thousand fare changes every month.

At one time mature travelers could even fly free on Northwest Airlines — provided they were 100 or older. Lately Northwest has promoted its club that offers 10 percent discounts to those 62 and over.

Mature travelers who shop for airfares often can get up to 50 percent off, depending on the day of travel and length of stay. America West recently quoted a Chicago-Las Vegas fare for seniors of only $65 — half off the lowest possible normal fare. And Southwest Airlines flies seniors anywhere in Texas and Razorback country for $19.

Eastern and Continental gave seniors one-third off all summer fares — $198 for a round-trip New York-Los Angeles ticket, $112 off. Seniors could fly round-trip Los Angeles-Orlando for only $200.

Some airlines, like Aloha, Braniff or Mexicana simply give seniors straight discounts on whatever ticket they buy. Southwest Airlines will fly anyone 65 and older to any of its Western cities for a flat $25 on most weekdays.

Other airlines make it complicated, with memberships and special passes and coupons required — but the savings always make the time spent applying for them worthwhile.

International airlines play the game, too: El Al had its deeply discounted "Milk 'N' Honey" promotion for seniors only during Israel's 40th anniversary.

Sabena offered a one-way "Discovery Fare" from New York to Brussels for travelers 60 and older at $169 — $80 off its lowest discount ticket for round trip. Finnair, TAP Air Portugal, LOT the Polish Airline and JAT Yugoslav Airlines all offer senior discounts of one kind or another.

One of the strangest was a Japan Air Lines offer in 1988 to fly married couples whose combined ages totaled 88 or more for 20 percent off.

SEASONS AND SITES FOR SENIORS

Some whole communities offer senior-citizen discounts, and, like all other senior citizen deals, they come and go quickly.

Colonial Williamsburg, Va., has "Senior Time" deals every September (Williamsburg Area Convention and Visitors Bureau, P.O. Box GB, Williamsburg, VA 23187). Orlando merchants and attractions, including Sea World and Cypress Gardens, organize special senior discounts from mid-September to mid-December (Greater Orlando Chamber of Commerce, P.O. Box 1234, Orlando, FL 32802).

Towns ranging from tiny Sierra Vista, Ariz., to Washington, D.C., sell senior travelers discount books with hundreds of coupons. And some entire countries, like Switzerland, woo seniors.

TOURS FOR SENIORS

The nice thing about tours for seniors is that the people who go on them are our age — no rambunctious kids, no teenagers with their noisy radios, no overachievers who just have to do Paris in one day and the rest of the world on the second day.

If you're a mature traveler taking a tour for seniors, you can be confident that there will be people on the tour just like you.

But that's not always desirable. *The Mature Traveler* newsletter tells about two ladies from Pittsburgh, both in their 60s, who told their travel agent that traveling with people just their own age was not their idea of a good time.

"We booked the main sitting," they told the editor, "and crossed our fingers we wouldn't be with other little old ladies." They weren't. They were seated for dinner with three couples, all on their honeymoons, and the little old ladies from Pittsburgh had a great time.

On the other hand, if you like to travel with people just like you, who'll keep the same pace you keep, who've grown up in the same era you did and who may even share many of your pleasures, you probably will enjoy trips that cater to older travelers.

Sometimes, too, your senior group will be temporarily mixed in with others — on a cruise, for example, or on a charter trip. So you'll have a chance to meet all kinds of people before your group goes on its own way.

Before you take a specially-advertised "tour for mature travelers," make sure it's something special. With some operators, all it stands for is that, "We'll take senior citizens' bucks along with everybody else's."

When you hear of a tour just for seniors, ask what makes it special. What features has it got just for you? Those features might range from discounts to safe-arrival phone calls. Here are some others:

• A mix of people limited to seniors — especially one that includes no young families with children.

• Itineraries that are broken into manageable pieces, without overnight flights or bus rides.

• Adventures that are within your physical ability. Try to avoid difficult adventures such as day-long walking tours of Venice, claustrophobic climbs to the burial chamber of the Great Pyramid and the like. Your Venice tour can be heavy on gondola sightseeing, and there's a lot of pleasure in viewing the Great Pyramid from the ground and hearing the lecture inside an air-conditioned motorcoach.

• Meals that avoid fats and salts.

• A cost structure that waives cancellation fees if you find at the last minute you can't go.

If you have to travel alone, look for tours that feature reduced single supplements—or none at all. (Most per-person hotel rates are based on double occupancy — two people to a room; a single supplement is an added price charged if you occupy a room by yourself. More about those in Chapter 2.)

A few tour organizations specialize in travel for senior citizens. Some of the largest ones are AARP, Grand Circle Travel and Saga Holidays. Since these tours are marketed directly to the public, and not through travel agents, you must write or phone them directly, and deal only with their travel counselors. All of these agencies offer worldwide trips as well as tours to the U.S. and Canada.

A very special tour packager is Grandtravel. It specializes in tours for grandparents traveling with their grandchildren. They've offered, for example, a spring-break visit to the Southwest to learn about American Indians, a Rose Bowl trip, a summer African Adventure Safari and a Crafts of Ireland tour.

Some European companies, such as Love Holidays and Amity Tours, incorporate things like folk-dance festivals and spa vacations in their trips for mature travelers. A list of travel packagers offering tours exclusively for seniors is at the end of this chapter.

JOINING SOMETHING

The best way to start taking advantage of senior-citizen travel bargains is to join something — whether you're a joiner or not. Join any of the thousands of clubs that earn travel discounts for their members.

One of the most popular is the American Automobile Association or one of its state affiliates. It has retail travel agencies at most of its offices, offers trip planning, provides several kinds of travel insurance and even takes care of towing your car if you're stuck in the countryside. In addition, AAA members get 10- to 20- percent discounts from Hertz, Avis and other car rentals; from Disneyland and many other amusement parks; from restaurants and motels and who knows what else?

The truth is that some travel-related companies, like the car rentals, will give you discounts whatever you belong to — AAA or any other auto club; Rotary, Kiwanis or any other service club; your college alumni club; your professional association; your credit union. These often are the same discounts they offer to members of seniors' clubs.

THOSE SENIORS' CLUBS

American Association of Retired Persons claims to be the largest club in the world, with the world's largest newspaper (in terms of circulation) and almost the world's largest magazine, *Modern Maturity*. If you have turned 50, you're eligible. For membership information, write AARP, 3200 E. Carson St., Lakewood, CA 90712.

While AARP doesn't bill itself as a travel club, one big benefit is package tours for its members — usually at special prices. It also negotiates member discounts. Its magazine and newsletter often have news of special travel deals for seniors. The annual membership fee is $5.

As a sampler, AARP membership will get you discounts at some major auto rental companies (10 to 25 percent off); Best Westerns, Econolodges, Holiday Inns, Howard Johnsons, Hospitality Internationals, Quality Internationals and Rodeway Inns; La Quintas and Sheratons (20 to 25 percent off); and Marriotts (up to half off).

Some other leading organizations, while not travel clubs, offer travel benefits similar to AARP's.

The National Council of Senior Citizens (925 15th St. N.W., Washington, DC 20005; ☎ phone 202/347-8800), for example, has no minimum age limit, though its average member is over 60. In addition to discounts at a range of domestic motels, the council has an unusual travel program incorporating low-cost resorts in Europe. Membership is $8 a year, $10 for couples.

Some companies that want to do business with senior citizens have started seniors' travel clubs. The biggest is Mature Outlook, a subsidiary of Sears, Roebuck & Co. and obviously formed to promote Sears' diverse products ranging from appliances to financial services — and travel. Like AARP, Mature Outlook packages tours for its members, who are 55 and over, and has a magazine. Dues are $7.50 a year. For membership information, contact any Sears store.

Another club typical of those with commercial connections is the September Days Club, a promotion of the Days Inn motel chain ☎ (toll-free 800/241-5050 for membership information). It provides member discounts on car rentals, on some airline tickets and, of course, at the chain's 300 or more motels. Many hotel chains and several airlines have similar seniors' travel clubs, and if there are no dues, what's the harm in joining, since you have to stay someplace, anyway?

There are all kinds of other travel clubs for seniors, including those sponsored by city recreation departments and senior-citizen centers.

There are special-interest groups, like the Catholic Golden Age Club, all offering some travel discounts for their members. Even your bank or savings and loan may sponsor a seniors' travel club.

All you have to do is ask.

IN SUMMARY

— A "senior citizen" can be any traveler over 45.
— The savvy mature traveler needn't pay full rate on anything.
— To find the best deals for mature travelers, subscribe to a good newsletter.
— Make sure your "senior-citizen" tour is really for seniors.
— Join clubs to get better mature traveler deals.

★ ★ ★
Travel Tool
★ ★ ★

TOURS FOR SENIORS

Here are some companies specializing in tours for mature travelers:

AARP Travel Service
— Tours for members through Olson-Travelworld. Budget trips, learning vacations, apartment stays, luxury tours and cruises almost everywhere. No travel agents. For catalogs, members only write P.O. Box 92337, Los Angeles, CA 90009; ☎ toll-free 800/227-7337.

Amity Tours
— Eastern Europe trips, including the Soviet Union, a specialty. Many tours for seniors feature mineral baths and treatments and folk-dancing demonstrations. Departure points can be from either U.S. coast. Book through your travel agent, or write for catalog to 2710 El Camino Real, Redwood City, CA 94063; ☎ toll-free 800/523-8406, in California 800/227-6928.

Elderhostel
— A program sponsored by colleges and other educational institutions for those 60 and over. It offers a low-cost educational trips throughout North America and abroad, with dormitory lodging on campuses. For course (tour) catalog, write 80 Boylston St. Suite 400, Boston, MA 02116; ☎ phone 617/426-8056.

50+ Young At Heart Travel Program
— Hosteling trips especially for mature travelers. American Youth Hostel Association, P.O. Box 37613, Washington, DC 20013-7613; ☎ phone 202/783-6161.

Golden Age Travellers
— Travel club format. Offers tours for seniors from West Coast points. No travel agents. For the club's newsletter and more information, write 1105 Taraval St., San Francisco, CA 94116; ☎ toll-free 800/258-8880, in California 800/652-1683.

Grand Circle Travel
— Offers a large number of escorted tours throughout the world exclusively for seniors, plus extended vacations. No travel agents. For brochures and catalogs, write 347 Congress St., Boston, MA 02210; ☎ toll-free 800/221-2610, in Massachusetts 800/535-8333.

Grandtravel
— Specializing in educational tours for grandparents and their grandchildren. No travel agents. Write The Ticket Counter, 6900 Wisconsin Ave., Chevy Chase, MD 20815; ☎ toll-free 800/247-76511.

Insight International
— Mostly deluxe motorcoach tours of Europe for those over 55. Book through travel agents or write for a catalog to P.O. Box 16247, Irvine, CA 92713; ☎ toll-free outside of California 800/952-9550.

Interhostel
— Sponsors a series of two-week international educational trips for travelers over 50. Write University of New Hampshire, 6 Garrison Ave., Durham, NH 03824; ☎ phone 603/862-1147.

Love Holidays
— Serves only the European market, including the Mediterranean, but with a U.S. office. This means you must get to European departure points on your own. But once you're there, prices are very competitive, and Love's tours earn good reviews. Book through your travel agent, or for catalog write 5530 Corbin Ave., Tarzana, CA 91356; ☎ toll-free outside of California 800/423-5458.

Mature Outlook
— Similar club format to AARP. Sponsored by Sears, Roebuck. Offers domestic, European and Orient tours for members only through Ask Mr. Foster travel agents. No local travel agents. For catalogs, write Mature Outlook, P.O. Box 1205, Glenview, IL 60025; ☎ phone 312/402-7800.

Mayflower Tours
— Designs tours especially for seniors, though it takes all ages. Offers motorcoach, plane and train trips throughout the U.S. and Canada, and cruises out of Florida ports. Book through your travel agent, or write P.O. Box 490, Downers Grove, IL 60515; ☎ toll-free 800/323-7604.

Passages Unlimited
— Offers world tours for mature travelers, as well as trips for single travelers and live-abroad packages. Check for tour offerings with your travel agent, or write 48 Union St., Stamford, CT 06906; ☎ phone toll-free 800/472-7724.

Saga Holidays
— British company with U.S. headquarters in Boston, claiming to be the largest travel company in the world for adults 60 and over. No travel agents. Write 120 Boylston St., Boston, MA 02116; ☎ toll-free 800/343-0273.

Senior Escorted Tours
— Trips for seniors from mid-Atlantic departure points. No travel agents. Write P.O. Box 400, Cape May Court House, NJ 08210; ☎ toll-free 800/222-1254, in New Jersey 800/222-1257.

Vistatours
— Offers selection of tours for seniors including trips with grandkids and special Festival of Roses party. Book through a travel agent or write 1923 N. Carson St., Suite 105 Carson City, NV 8971; ☎ toll-free 800/647-0800 or 702/882-2100.

Yugotours
— For retirees or anyone over 59. Moderately priced tours from U.S. to Yugoslavia and nearby destinations like Greece, Egypt, Russia, Austria, Italy. Book through a travel agent, or write 350 Fifth Ave. Suite 2212, New York, NY 10118; ☎ toll-free 800/223-5298, in New York 212/563-2400.

CHAPTER 2

MAKING YOUR DREAM TRIP COME TRUE — WITHOUT HASSLE

| The Better You Plan, The Better Your Trip Will Be |

O nce you get an itch to travel, you've got to scratch it. And once you start scratching, you may never stop.

If you're retired, you've got the time to plan your trips and choose the very best opportunities to go. You can do a lot of armchair traveling before you actually start on your dream trip.

On the other hand, you've also got the flexibility to travel whenever you feel like it — to take a long weekend at a golf resort if the right discount pops up; to hop in the car or the RV and spend a week in the mountains when it gets too warm at home; to take a short cruise just for a change of scenery.

And you've also probably got more money to spend on travel than you ever had before, now that the kids are gone and house and car are paid for. Besides, travel is getting to be less expensive — for seniors more than most. That dream trip now is within reach of almost every mature traveler.

The big problem is the wide range of choices for your dream trip — a ride on the Orient Express or barging through England; a drive through the Rockies or driving down to Disney World; a winter getaway to the Caribbean or a Baja fishing trip; or a weekend in the wine country, in Quebec, or in the Ozarks? Shall you take a guided tour or explore on your own? Should you talk to a travel agent, or plan it yourself? Do you want to go just with other seniors, or do young people get your juices moving? And how do you know how much to spend on your dream trip? After all, you can take a lot of dream trips if you plan them right.

What is your dream trip, anyhow? Was it the one you've just taken — or the trip that still lies ahead?

Whichever — start thinking about it now.

PLANNING YOUR DREAM TRIP

The more carefully you plan your travel, the more fun you'll have traveling.

The planning process — time-consuming only if you want it to be — is simple:

1) Writing down where you'd like to go.
2) Determining when you can go.
3) Figuring out how much you want to spend.
4) Choosing how you want to go.

We are not about to tell you where to go or how to get there. Travel is a personal thing.

Just because your friends had a good trip somewhere, doesn't mean you will, too. You might appreciate a museum in Chicago more than the horse races in England. Or a visit to Pearl Harbor more than snorkeling at Molokini. Some people travel to get away from friends and relatives — others travel to visit them. If you hate to fly, your dream trips should be around the United States, Mexico and Canada, no matter how much your friends enjoyed Spain. If you know you get seasick, forget that seven-day cruise to five Caribbean ports — you won't like it, even if Uncle Joe did have the time of his life.

On the other hand, most travelers have a big curiosity bump. You know there's a lot of walking and climbing to get to Machu-Picchu, but the photos make it look so serene up there . . . . You might get seasick, but how do you know until you try a short cruise to Catalina and the Baja?

Some travelers' tastes run to an African photo-safari; some others' to a visit to the Ice Hockey Hall of Fame in Ely, Minn. So, for a start, you must figure out where your own tastes might take you.

Then make a list: 20, maybe 30, trips you want to take — short ones and long ones. Just think about them. Do a little reading on some of the places, if you want. Finally, focus on the next year or two and get your list down to a manageable half-a-dozen or fewer.

If you're a decisive person, it's even simpler:

Just say, "Darnit, I've always wanted to go to (fill in the blank), and now I'm going to do it!" And your list is down to one.

TIMING YOUR TRIP

If you're still working, you may be locked into a company vacation schedule. Or you may have to attend an upcoming family reunion. Maybe you have tickets for the 49ers-Redskins game that you're not going to give up for any reason. These kinds of things help you determine when to travel.

If you're self-employed or retired, on the other hand, you can probably go almost any time, and the question becomes: when do you want to travel? Here are some considerations that might help you decide:

• The seasons — To get there when the weather is at its very best, it makes sense to go south in the winter, north in the summer. These are the "high seasons. " Here are dates for some of the customary "high seasons" at popular tourist destinations:

Hawaii, the Caribbean, Mexico and Florida, Dec. 15-April 15. Desert Southwest, January through April. The American West, June through Labor Day. Europe, June through early October. Ski resorts, Dec. 15-March 31.

• The crowds — High seasons are the times when everybody else will be going, too. Wherever you go in the summer, in fact, you'll run into schoolkids and mobs of people; there'll be lines at major attractions, and restaurant service will be slow. But in the "shoulder months" of April-May and September-October, the kids are back in school and the crowds thin out — besides, the weather will be almost as good, though you'll be taking a little more chance.

• The cost — In popular tourist areas, high seasons are the most expensive, low season the least. Some areas also have transition prices. In areas where there's a high season and the weather is extreme, the savings are astounding when you travel off-season. In Palm Springs and Tucson and other Southwest locations, resorts that regularly get $200-$250 per room will rent you one for $40-$50 in the off-season. You'll get wonderful golf deals and half-price attractions. And you can beat the heat by getting up at dawn to fish or golf nine holes, spend days in an air-conditioned museum or in the shade beside a pool, nap in the afternoon and then catch another nine holes just before the sun goes down.

• Local conditions — Whatever the season, rooms and restaurant reservations can be impossible to get whenever a big local event is going on: Mardi Gras in New Orleans for example, or when the American Legion convention is in town. Once we were literally rushed out of Munich the morning before Oktoberfest was to begin without even time for a beer — they needed our rooms.

If you're attending one of these events, fine — no doubt your travel agent or the organizing committee will have reserved a big block of rooms. But otherwise, these are good times to avoid. If you can get reservations at all, you'll pay dearly.

If you're nervous about the timing of your trip, write the local tourist agencies for calendars of events, local holidays and climate information (see Chapter 4) or ask your travel agent for advice.

BUDGETING YOUR TRIP

Some readers always ask how much per day they should spend on a trip. And we usually reply, "What trip?"

Rules of thumb are misleading — but if you have to have some, we think any trip under $100 a day per person is a real bargain. For any trip that budgets out more than $200 a day, we try to find corners to cut or another way to get there.

A package tour — and there are many good ones — will be cheaper than a similar tour you plan yourself. But it may include things you don't really want to see.

Instead of a travel "bargain," look for a travel "value. "

That depends on where you're going and when and how and in what style. You could visit Kalamazoo, Mich. , for a lot less than $100 a day — that doesn't make it a bargain. A ride on the Orient Express costs more than $1,000 a day — but we'd guess there are more than 10 times the thrills on the train, which makes the Orient Express a travel value. We should add, "in our view." If you suffer acute motion sickness, you'll probably disagree.

Approach travel budgeting as an approximation — a ballpark estimate. At the start of your planning session, know what your personal budget allows for travel. You don't have to spend it all for one trip, but make a rough allocation, something like this:

"We're going to take four short trips this year at $500 each, and two major trips at $3,000 each. "

These are figures to shoot at, to figure out whether your dream trip is practical now, or whether you'll have to scale down your plans and save some travel for next year. Maybe you have a little give, also — you can cut out a couple of the short trips, or get by with a single major trip, if it's a great one.

Thus, you come up with a ballpark figure for your trip — in this example, $3,000 to $5,000. That's a figure to give your travel agent as a "budget," or to play around with if you're planning your own trip.

It may not be a practical budget for the trip you want to take: $3,000 will get you less than a week in Tokyo, for example, unless you swim to get there. But that budget might last three weeks or more in Acapulco.

One way to see how far your budget will stretch is to try it out against this table put out by the U. S. State Department. For various cities, the department computes the cost for two people traveling together and staying at a moderately priced hotel, eating three meals daily. It includes incidentals and local transportation, but not airfare getting there. Figures are for late 1988:

For two people to stay in:	The daily cost is:
Acapulco	$114
Amsterdam	243
Aruba	277
Athens	160
Bali	186
Bangkok	184
Barbados	228
Buenos Aires	162
Cancún	228

Dublin	346
Hong Kong	308
London	365
Madrid	268
Melbourne	217
Mexico City	141
New York	258
Orlando	150
Paris	369
Rio de Janeiro	213
Stockholm	331
Tel Aviv	209
Tokyo	460
Toronto	213
Venice	325

A more accurate way to see how far your budget will take you is to cost out your dream trip. Write or use toll-free phone numbers to get airfares, brochures, directories, guides and rough prices for everything (see Chapter 4, Armchair Travel). Then add up the costs. Use the form "Figuring Your Travel Budget" at the end of this chapter.

And if you're doing your own planning, rather than using a travel agent, it should also become the master plan for your dream trip.

IF YOUR BUDGET DOESN'T WORK

Don't give up your dream trip just because you're short of cash. One way to make up the difference is to put off the trip for a little while until you can save the difference — and do that systematically: figure out how much you need and set aside a fixed amount every month marked "Travel" until you can afford to go.

Some travelers simply go now and pay later — using credit cards heavily, or even taking out a loan. That's OK if it's your trip-of-a-lifetime. But you might find it demoralizing planning next year's big trip while you're still trying to pay for this year's. Here are some better ways to make your travel dollar stretch a little further:

Take a group tour. Have your travel agent try to find a tour that's close to matching your dream trip.

Travel off-season. You won't have to pay premium rates.

Get a budget guidebook to help you to find less expensive restaurants, hotels, day-tours.

Scale down your lodgings. Use hostels, for example. Look for a home swap, or a "catered" apartment (see Chapter 5, Lodging).

Stay in small towns or the countryside, then day-trip into larger cities. Lodgings and meals will be a cheaper, and the pace more relaxed.

Plan on using buses and subways instead of taxis, and buy unlimited- use passes for public transit in European cities.

Ask for the senior-citizen discount wherever you go, here or abroad. Sometimes, you can save up to 50 percent on hotels, 25 percent on meals (see Chapter 5, Lodging).

KINDS OF TOURS

Wherever you want to go, there are a hundred ways to get there. You can arrange the trip yourself or work through a travel agent. Either way, you can travel independently, take an escorted tour or a package tour on your own. If you want to go with a special group, you can take a tour just for seniors, a tour for RVers (recreational vehicle users), a tour for auto fans, a golf tour and so on.

Cruiseships have jazz tours, bridge tours, square-dance tours, archaeological tours, ballet tours . . . the list is endless. You can even take a mix-and-match tour: fly/drive Europe, fly/cruise the Far East, motorcoach/cruise the U. S. southeast coast; cruise the Caribbean and stop at Disney World.

To add to the confusion, tour operators can also act as travel agencies, and retail travel agents sometimes put together tours. Of course, you can just buy your ticket or hop in your car and go.

Here are some organized ways to travel:

Independent travel — Tour agents call it FIT (for "foreign independent travel"). It can be the most expensive, and also the most rewarding, way to go. You or your travel agent tailor a trip just for you.

Group tours — Though there are few senior discounts available on these, they are less expensive because they can take advantage of group rates and mass consumption. If a tour operator who runs weekly trips to Jamaica for 100 people in the winter can book 2,000 hotel rooms all at once, or 2,000 airline seats, he will get a very good rate, indeed. And he passes part of the savings along to his customers in the tour price.

A group tour also relieves you of the details of planning a trip, and provides companions to share the joys of the trip.

On the downside, because the tour itinerary is set, you go only where the group goes and do what the group does. To offset that, most tour itineraries provide some free time — the more free time, the more flexible the tour.

There are different kinds of tours with different degrees of freedom — fully escorted, hosted, independent and so on. Though tour operators describe them in different ways, the generally accepted meanings of those terms are at the end of this chapter.

For some trips, you have to take group tours — to most Iron Curtain countries, for example, or to Tibet, where many religious sites are restricted. For other trips, it just makes savings and good sense — especially if you're a gregarious type who likes to share travel adventures with others.

Make sure the tour company is a reputable one. Quiz your travel agent, or get the names of other travelers in your area who have taken the tour and phone them to find out if they were satisfied. Read the tour brochure carefully, including the asterisks and the fine print (see Chapter 4, Armchair Travel). Make sure the tour includes what you've been told it includes. Especially, find out what happens to your money if the tour is canceled.

One test of a tour company is how long it's been in business. Those who run inferior tours don't last long. Another good indication of reliability is membership in the United States Tour Operators Association (USTOA) or American Society of Travel Agents (ASTA). USTOA members have to carry liability insurance and post a bond against any disputes. You can write USTOA for a list of its members at 211 E. 51st St. , New York, NY 10022.

ASTA can take formal action against its members if they violate the organization's code of ethics, and you can write to find out whether there are any unresolved complaints against an operator — P. O. Box 23992, Washington, DC 20026-3992; ☎ phone 703/739-2782.

Tour packages — Even if you're an independent traveler, don't turn up your nose at tour packages. They can save you money. Yes, some packages can add up to full tours. But most simply combine two or more elements of a vacation you'd take anyway — lodging and golf, for example. And the discounts you get from buying a tour package are sometimes as good as those on group tours.

A fly/drive Hawaii package, for example, includes airfare and a rental car — perhaps a hotel is part of the package, too. But that in no way restricts your freedom to go where you want and see what you want to see. Fly/cruise packages are common. Ski weekends that include lodging, maybe some meals and lift tickets, are kinds of tour packages.

The joy of these is that you get group rates, but you don't have to be with the group.

BEATING THE SINGLES SUPPLEMENTS

Those who travel together almost always go cheaper than solo travelers. The culprit is called the "single supplement," and it's particularly tough on mature travelers.

Tour operators usually add a few hundred dollars to the price for singles, because they assume you'll be staying in a cabin or at an inn by yourself. At hotels and motels, singles pay a 50 percent penalty — or higher. And on cruises the cost for traveling alone is sometimes double — when one person pays the same price as two for a cabin.

And despite the higher cost, a single often winds up in a pie-shaped room behind the elevator, or in a tiny cabin near the galley.

The number of solo travelers — whether widowed or by choice — has increased by 12-to-15 percent in the past five years, according to Cruise Lines International Association, and most of these travelers are 49ers-plus.

The only sure ways to avoid these high single supplements are to find a traveling companion or take a singles trip or cruise.

TRAVEL-PARTNER CLUBS

To help you find a travel companion, there are hundreds of travel-partner clubs around the country, many just for 49ers-plus. Most of them charge an annual or semi-annual fee, have you fill out a questionnaire (personal habits, your travel tastes, where you want to go and the like) and publish it in a regular newsletter for members. It's up to you to contact other club members you're interested in traveling with.

Most travel-partner clubs are local. The best place to find one is the classified section of your local newspaper or through a senior-citizens center.

The advantage of arranging your own travel partner is that you can correspond in advance, get to match tastes and travel habits or get a chance to search for another partner if the first one turns out to be incompatible.

Here are some nationwide clubs that serve 49ers-plus:

Golden Companions — Limited to single travelers 50 and over. Based in Northwest U. S. P. O. Box 754, Pullman, WA 99163. Members get bi-monthly newsletter with new-member listings, travel companion ads. Also offers discounts on tours promoted by A. J. S. Travel Consultants in New York, which specializes in trips for seniors.

Partners In Travel — President Miriam Tobolowsky says she's "the grandma of travel partners clubs," having founded this one in 1981. For $40/year ($25/6 months) members get a bimonthly newsletter with up to 200 want-ads per issue. The club provides ID numbers for advertisers and forwards replies. About 90 percent of the club's 700 members are 49ers-plus. P. O. Box 491145, Los Angeles, CA 90049.

Travel Companion Exchange — Largest club in the country, with members nationwide. Large majority are 49ers-plus. It's been operating since 1983. Current semi-yearly dues are $66 — but only $36 if you're looking for a partner of the same sex. Send in your form and you get the current *Weekly Advanced List* of new members and those actively looking. You also get back issues of *Travel Companions*, a bimonthly newsletter, which will list all members. The club does not offer box numbers — you contact members directly. P. O. Box 833, Amityville, NY 11701; ☎ 516/454-0880.

Travel Share International — Club provides a bi-monthly directory with personal profiles of the members and their travel goals. Dues vary. P. O. Box 30365, Santa Barbara, CA 93130. ☎ 805/965-9455.

SINGLES TOURS

Almost any travel agency can book a singles tour for you. Some tour operators put you up with roommates; others let you stay alone and just charge a little more. The joy of the latter is that you've got a whole group of traveling companions to enjoy traveling with, and also a place to be alone when you want to be. That may be worth the extra expense.

While some singles tours are great for mature travelers, many such tours are for youngsters who want to romp. And you can't always tell them apart until you look at the brochures. Singleworld, for example, advertises two kinds of tours: "All age groups" and "under-35 groups." If that's not a clue, their brochure is: it shows only young people at play. On the other hand, even if you didn't know that Grand Circle Travel caters only to 49ers-plus, the photos in its brochures would give you that message.

Before you sign up for a singles tour, ask your travel agent, "Who goes on these things?" And if the answer contradicts the photos in the brochure, forget it.

Both Saga Holidays ☎ 800/669-7242 and Grand Circle Travel ☎ 800/221-2100 specialize in trips for mature travelers. Saga sometimes has singles-only departures of their regular tours, though they charge the regular single supplement. Even so, their single supplements are among the lowest we've seen — usually less than 10 percent. While Grand Circle doesn't have singles-only tours, like Saga, it offers to match you up with a travel partner or reduce the single-hotel-room supplement by 50 percent. On some tours, both Saga and Grand Circle waive the single supplement.

GUARANTEE PROGRAMS

Some cruiselines and tour operators have guaranteed-share programs for singles. You pay only the per-person double-occupancy rate, and the promoter tries to match you with a suitable roommate. And there are variations on that plan: American Express requires you to pay the single supplement up-front, but gives you a refund if they can find a travel partner.

The drawback with these plans is that you have little choice who you're matched with — and an incompatible roommate can spoil a trip.

TRIP INSURANCE

What happens to your advance payment if you become ill and can't take the trip? How can you get your money back if the tour operator goes broke or cancels your trip? What if you lose your luggage overseas and have to buy new clothes? What if you have to come home in the middle of the trip, and have to pay additional airfare?

No problem — the insurance company will pay for most of it. You can get insurance, you know, against almost any calamity. If you worry a lot, investigate getting extra trip insurance for your peace of mind.

Trip-cancellation insurance is sold directly by insurance companies, or through travel agents. It's not cheap — often running more than 5 percent of the insured amount. Of course, you don't need insurance for the whole cost of the trip — only for the extra amount you'd be out should the trip be canceled, perhaps just any advance payments you've made.

A typical policy is sold by Travel Guard International. It pays any extra expenses you incur, including loss of advance payments, if your trip is called off as a result of death, injury, illness, a strike, supplier default — even jury duty.

Some companies handling trip-cancellation insurance are:

Access America, 600 Third Ave. , Box 807, New York, NY 10163 ☎ 800/284-8300.

Travel Guard International, 1100 Center Point Dr. , Stevens Point, WI 54481 ☎ 800/826-1300.

Tele-Trip Co. , 3201 Farnam St. , Omaha, NE 68131

☎ 800/228-9792.

WorldCare Travel Assistance Assn. , 2000 Pennsylvania Ave. N.W., Suite 7600, Washington, DC 20006 ☎ 800/521-4822.

Extra medical insurance for your trip also is available from Access America, a division of Blue Cross-Blue Shield, and a number of other leading medical insurers. They're described and listed in Chapter 20, To Your Health.

You can buy special baggage insurance, life insurance and auto insurance, too. But you may already have enough insurance against travel calamity. Does your homeowners' or renters' policy cover that lost luggage or a stolen wallet? How well does your auto insurance cover that rental car abroad? Check with your own insurance agent before you buy a costly extra policy.

As for those quickie life-insurance policies you can buy from vending machines at airports, forget it. For one thing, they're tremendously overpriced. For another, the credit card company you charged your ticket to probably already has you covered for the trip. And you have your own life insurance, too — is your life worth any more in the air than it is on the ground?

For any kind of coverage, a good rule is never over-insure. Consider how much loss you can take care of yourself, and insure for anything over that amount.

ASSISTANCE INSURANCE

Becoming more available for American travelers is "assistance insurance" — insurance that gets you the help you need in a personal emergency, as well as the money.

Perhaps you need an English-speaking doctor, legal help, a bail bond, an emergency airlift. Assistance insurance policies provide you with local telephone numbers where you can get fast help almost anywhere in the world, in addition to the usual medical benefits, emergency cash and the like. Typical prices range from $15 a person for a one-week trip, to $200 for a family for a year, depending on the kinds of protection provided.

Like other kinds of travel insurance, you can buy an assistance policy from your travel agent, or direct from the insurer. Three companies selling Assistance policies are:

Access America (see section on trip insurance).

Europe Assistance Worldwide Services, Inc., 1333 F St. N.W., Suite 300, Washington, DC 20004; ☎ toll free 800/821-2828.

International SOS Assistance, Inc. , Box 11568, Philadelphia, PA. 19116; ☎ toll-free 800/523-8930.

THE FINAL PLAN

Now you've got a timetable, a budget and some rough ideas on where and how you'd like to go.

If you don't plan to involve a travel agent at this point, or to take a cruise or an escorted tour, get all the literature you can for the half-dozen places on your final list (see Chapter 4, Armchair Travel, for sources of information).

Start with magazine articles from your public library on the places you want to visit. Read guidebooks about each place — by then you probably will have narrowed your choices to one or two dream trips. Buy the guidebooks at your local bookstore, or borrow them from your public library.

Then begin detail planning. Get lists of inns and prices, maps of the region, transportation schedules, lists of events and attractions — Chapter 4 tells you where to write. Make your own list of things you'd like to do and see.

Get a calendar and plan what you'd like to do each day of your trip. Plan where you'll stay and, if possible, where you'd like to eat. Map your route if it's a driving trip, and make advance reservations for the first night or two out — motels fill up fast in the summer.

To avoid long lines and disappointments, make reservations for lodging and any special side-trips — like rafting or backpacking — as far in advance as you can. If there's a famous restaurant where you want to eat, make an advance reservation there, too. If you're a golfer, you'll need to get tee-times at least three weeks in advance at most major resorts. Use your credit card instead of your checkbook whenever you can to guarantee advance reservations — that way, you're sure of getting your money back if you cancel.

Think through every detail, and you'll begin to realize that planning a good trip takes some work — but the pleasure of traveling will be worth every bit of that effort.

IN SUMMARY:

— Planning steps are dreaming about the places you want to go; figuring when you can go, budgeting, paring your dream list to a single place and filling in the details.

— Look for travel value, not just bargains.

— Traveling with someone else is always less expensive than traveling alone.

— If your budget doesn't work, don't give up the trip; just find some corners to cut.

— Don't overspend on travel insurance.

★ ★ ★
Travel Tool
★ ★ ★

PLANNING YOUR TRAVEL BUDGET

Here are common vacation expenses. After you collect brochures, guidebooks and transportation fares, use this table to figure the approximate cost of your dream trip. Then see whether you can afford it. Use this computation, also, to compare one trip against another:

Common Travel Expenses	Estimated Cost
Transportation:	
Air/train/bus	_____
Airport bus	_____
Taxi(s)	_____
Parking	_____
Car or RV rental	_____
Gasoline	_____
Tolls	_____
Boat charter	_____
Tour (basic price)	_____
Cruise (basic price)	_____
Food and Lodging:	
Accommodations	_____
Meals/snacks	_____

Activities:
    Special equipment   _____
    Entertainment/sports   _____
    Equipment rental   _____
    Guided tours/excursions   _____
    Lessons   _____

Miscellaneous:
    Immunizations   _____
    Passport/visa(s)   _____
    New luggage   _____
    New clothes   _____
    Film/development   _____
    Other tips   _____
    Shopping/gifts   _____

Other: _____

Subtotal	_____
Plus 5% (for unexpected costs)	_____
Total	_____
Budget available	_____
Shortage, if any	_____

Divide by amount I can save monthly   _____
Months before I can take my dream trip   _____

Table courtesy of the money Management Institute of Household Financial Services, Prospect Heights, Illinois.

★ ★ ★
Travel Tool
★ ★ ★

TERMS YOU SHOULD KNOW

Here are some definitions of terms used in the travel industry that will help you understand what the brochures mean when you're planning your dream trip:

All-Inclusive Tour — A fully-escorted tour that includes transportation, lodging, most meals, sightseeing, transfers and most tips — almost all the expenses of your trip except personal ones like drinks, laundry, shopping and the like. Read the fine print and material behind the asterisks to find out what isn't included. Look for the letter "O" (for "optional"), which means that an item will cost extra.

APEX Fare — APEX stands for "Advance Purchase Excursion. " International airlines give you discounts for purchasing tickets well in advance of your flight — usually 60 days or more.

Baggage Allowance — The weight, size or number of bags that may be carried by an air passenger without extra charge. The allowance varies by airline, airplane and whether you're traveling domestically or overseas.

Bucket Shop — Travel agency that specializes in last-minute travel discounts, especially cruises and other tours. Last-minute travel clubs are examples.

Charter — Tour on which all individuals are on the same itinerary. Package can be air transportation alone, or can include lodgings or other land arrangements.

Connecting Flight — A segment of an ongoing trip that requires a change of planes, though not necessarily a change of airlines.

Direct Flight — A flight on which passengers don't have to change planes, but will have one or more stops en route.

Driver-Guide — Professional who drives a tour vehicle and points out places of interest.

Drop-Off Charge — An extra fee charged by a car rental company when you leave the car someplace other than where you got it.

Escorted Tour — A tour accompanied throughout by the same tour director, who stays at your hotel and is available for advice and planning.

FIT — Foreign Independent Tour is one on which you're traveling in a foreign country on your own, rather than with a group. Usually the most expensive way to travel abroad.

Force Majeure — An event, like a riot or an earthquake, that cannot be reasonably anticipated or controlled.

Full-Service Agency — A travel agency that can provide any service a traveler typically needs. Less-than-full-service agencies write just airline tickets, or specialize in commercial travel, cruise travel, limited geographical areas and the like.

Gateway Cities — Points of departure for tours and cruiselines' air supplements, whether domestic or overseas. Also, the last city of departure or the first city of arrival in international travel.

Group Inclusive Tour (GIT) — You get a group rate on a plane, though you don't have to travel with the group once you arrive. These are often sold with a land package. A minimum stay may be required.

High-Season Supplement — Additional charge for a tour or lodging during the busiest time of the year.

Hosted Tour — A tour that uses local hosts at each major destination to conduct local sightseeing and advise tour members on independent plans.

Hotel Categories — Deluxe, first-class, moderate and tourist-class are generally the descriptions used, though standards vary from country to country. You may want to stay away from any hotel less than first-class. For detailed descriptions, see Chapter 5, Lodging.

Hotel Plans — American, Continental, European or Modified American. See Chapter 5, Lodging.

Independent Tour — "Carefree," "Freelance," whatever. Tour operators have different names for this plan. These are unhosted package tours — you are on your own to explore, though a representative of the company is usually available to book sightseeing trips or answer questions.

Land Price — The portion of cost of a tour that includes land arrangements only, not transportation to the site where the tour begins.

Local Guide — Professional who conducts tours of specific locations and attractions.

Local Host — A representative of the tour operator who provides information and arranges sightseeing and entertainment in a particular city.

Non-Stop Flight — A direct flight between two points without any stops en route.

No-Shows — Those with reservations who don't show up.

Overbooking — The practice of selling too many seats or too many rooms with the expectation that some travelers will cancel or not show up.

Passport — An official government document certifying citizenship and granting permission to travel abroad.

Single Supplement — Premium added to tour or cruise price for a person traveling alone.

Tour Director — The tour escort or tour manager, who stays with a group for the whole tour.

Tour Operator — Or wholesaler. The creator of a travel package usually sold through travel agents.

Tourist Hotel (also Economy or Second Class) — A budget hotel with limited services and few private baths.

Transfers — Arrival and departure service, including transportation from airport, pier or rail station to hotel and baggage handling.

Visa — A government authorization appended to a passport permitting travel within a particular country.

Vouchers — Documents issued by tour operators to be exchanged for lodgings or other services. Substitute for cash payments.

NOTES

CHAPTER 3

YOUR FRIEND, THE TRAVEL AGENT

A Good One Can Save You a Bundle

Instead of doing all the work yourself, visit a travel agent. It rarely costs you a dime, and a good travel agent can save you a bundle. That's because travel agents earn their commissions from the airlines, hotels and tour packagers where they send you.

Usually the only thing a travel agent will charge you for is long-distance phone calls, extraordinary time-consuming research you ask for or other special services.

A full-service travel agent can sort through an enormous amount of information and come up with more vacation options — and at better prices — than you ever could yourself. A travel agent can warn you of potholes in your path, and find hidden roses behind the rocks. A good travel agent counsels you, takes an interest in making your trip successful and becomes your friend.

HOW TO SELECT AN AGENT

The best way to select a travel agency is the recommendation of a friend who's had a good trip. Otherwise, look in the Yellow Pages.

A few agencies specialize — some in business travel, some in ethnic travel, some in cruise travel, some in specific destinations like the Far East or the Caribbean. Full-service agencies — large or small — mostly have access to the same information, the

45

same fares and the same tours as the specialists, though their individual travel counselors may not be as familiar with the specialty.

If you've already decided on a cruise, go to a cruise specialist by all means. Otherwise, try to find a full-service agency that can offer more options.

Make sure the agency you select has a computer — one of the standard data-base systems that gives agents access to schedules, fares, hotels and other information and permits them to write airline tickets. And make sure the agency is a member of the American Society of Travel Agents (ASTA) or the Association of Retail Travel Agents (ARTA) — simply look for the plaques on the walls.

Whether you go to a big agency or a small one doesn't make that much difference. Though huge agencies with multiple branches — like Ask Mr. Foster, AAA World Travel or American Express — have more travel counselors, your odds of finding a good one there are just about the same as at a smaller agency.

If you're still in the browsing stage, collecting information on various places you might want to see, simply visit the largest agency you can find and ask for some ideas. Don't take up a lot of the agent's time, because they don't earn commissions just passing out brochures. If you think you want to cruise the Caribbean, pick up literature from half-a-dozen different cruiselines that serve the area regularly; if you want to go to Russia, pick up brochures on four or five different escorted tours.

If you've got a firmer idea of where you're going and are ready for some serious planning, it's time to sit down with a travel counselor and discuss your destination, your budget and your timing. If you know the manager or the owner, go to that person first. Chances are you'll get superb treatment from whatever counselor he refers you to, once it's known the boss is interested in your trip.

You don't have to do business with the first travel counselor you sit down with. Ask to talk to someone who's familiar with the area you want to visit, who's actually been there and has some contacts there. You won't find a specialist in every area of the world at every agency. But you can expect direct knowledge of popular destinations like London, Hawaii, France and so on.

Any trainee at a travel agency can organize a routine trip that involves writing airline tickets, putting you up at a hotel within your budget and arranging sightseeing. But if this is your trip-of-a-lifetime (or even your trip-of-the-year), you want to talk to someone with more experience. Ask to see a Certified Travel Counselor — one with the initials "C.T.C." on his business card. This person will be a travel pro, one who has traveled, who has at least five years' experience as a travel agent and who has completed graduate-level studies offered by the Institute of Certified Travel Agents in Wellesley, Mass.

If you know you're going to be taking other trips, too, try to establish a personal relationship, so the travel counselor will know your preferences, your budget and the kind of traveler you are — even alert you to a trip that's coming up if it's the kind you like.

WHAT A TRAVEL AGENT DOES

You arrive tired in a strange city where they speak a strange language, and the hotel has never heard of you, even though you've got a written confirmation. You can't call your travel agent because it's half-way around the world and the office is closed. By the time you sort things out by yourself, you'll swear your travel agent is a no-good bum.

Then there's the other kind of story: once we'd gotten a car in Dijon, and less than four blocks from where we'd picked it up, the engine blew up. We walked back to the auto-rental office, keys in hand, crying something like, "L'auto — il fait poof — poof!" Apparently "poof" is not a universal word for explosion. Nobody there spoke English; clearly, we didn't do French. But our travel counselor had given us the name of an English-speaking friend in Paris — another travel counselor who could sort out any problem, he said.

We whipped out the phone number, gestured toward the telephone and had the office clerk call for help. Our Paris contact translated, and within five minutes we had a new car and were on our way again. It worked that way throughout a fairly complicated journey — no missed connections, no screwups despite a last-minute change in itinerary and nice little touches everywhere. By the time we got back, we could swear our travel counselor was a miracle worker.

Travel counselors aren't, really — they're just professionals with all grades of skill. When *Money* magazine asked 10 different travel agencies to plan a trip to London, they came up with almost identical itineraries ranging in price from $697 to $1,131.

"We found an annoying number of uninformed travel agents, a distressing range of prices and frequently slipshod follow-through," *Money* reported, concluding that:

"A crack agent will design a custom itinerary or assemble parts or all of the best pre-arranged tours. A hack agent will go with the first wholesaler he can get through to on the phone, or the one who spirited him off on his last junket. In either case, the commissions are 8 percent to 10 percent."

Some of the things you can expect a travel agent to do for you include planning the best, least-expensive trip possible that meets the budget, timetable and requirements you specify; to arrange transportation, lodging, sightseeing, auto rentals, admission to theaters, meals at leading restaurants; to put you in the hands of reliable tour operators; to give you advice on things like clothes, the weather, tipping, health and money matters; to make all reservations you need, get all the tickets and vouchers, provide a written itinerary and written confirmations everywhere; to sell you insurance for lost baggage, trip cancellation or medical problems abroad; to handle any paperwork like passport and visa applications; to give you a safety net if something goes wrong — some place to call, some person to see.

In return, you have to be honest with your agent about your tastes and your budget, have some firm ideas about the kind of trip you want to take, and be ready to make advance deposits and pay bills when the agent calls for them.

The agent's not even done when you get home. If you've had trouble on the trip, call on the agent for help sorting out disputes and getting refunds. It will help, of course, if you've kept receipts, detailed notes on the problem and the names of people you talked to.

Even if you haven't had any problems, thank your travel agent. The good agents like to hear details of your trip and get feedback — it will help the next client they serve.

DISCOUNT TRAVEL AGENTS

If you already know what trip or cruise you want, discount travel agencies can save you money. They won't provide any research or customized service — that's up to you. And while they'll save you big money on a big trip, they'll save almost nothing on a two-hour flight.

Discounters, relying on big volume, rebate you part of their commissions. They typically sell tickets, tours and cruises at face value, then send back rebate checks usually amounting to 8-to-11 percent of the ticket price, less a handling fee — and up to 25 percent on international flights.

McTravel Travel Services in Chicago ☎ toll-free 800/333-3335, one of the biggest discounters, charges handling fees ranging from $25 (for bookings under $1,000) to $50 (over $1,000). Recent savings quoted by McTravel range from only $4 on a Minneapolis-Dallas round-trip flight, to $38 on the Orient Express, and $96 on Eastern Airline's senior Get Up and Go Passport. McTravel would save you approximately $450 on a $5,000 cruise. You don't have to live in Chicago to use McTravel.

There are discount agencies in almost every major city, and most of them have toll-free 800 numbers. Watch for their ads in travel sections of local newspapers.

A consolidators is a special kind of discounter who buys blocks of unsold seats, cruiseship cabins and hotel rooms at deep discounts, and passes part of the savings along to the traveler. Their rates are usually even better than the discounters'. But it's hard to plan ahead to use a consolidator — their deals come and go quickly. Watch for their ads, too, in local newspapers.

LAST-MINUTE TRAVEL CLUBS

The very best deals in travel are for those whose time is flexible — who can go whenever the tour goes, and who can get ready on very short notice. These last-minute travel clubs, while they're open to everyone, are especially good for retired people who aren't tied to a work schedule and who live near major departure points.

The deals these clubs offer are based on "the empty-seat theory" — that a seat filled at any price is better than an empty one. These are regularly scheduled tours, not cheapies. And you get confirmed reservations, not standbys.

It works this way: Tour packagers have to make commitments in advance — so many airline tickets, so many hotel rooms, so much tour-bus space and the like. Tour operators pay a guaranteed wholesale price for the accommodations, package them and sell them to the public at something less than retail. But if a seat is unsold, the packager still has to pay for it.

To make sure that doesn't happen, packagers will sell their unsold seats at last-minute prices. The packager can't advertise those unsold seats at discount prices, though, because those who've paid full-ticket would want a rebate.

So the packager hands the unsold seats to discount travel clubs — travel clearinghouses that have lists of people who have already indicated they can travel almost on call. If you're on the list, you'll get opportunities to save 10 to 70 percent on travel to some very nice places. But to take advantage of them, you have to be flexible: you may get only two weeks' notice or less.

Here's a recent typical deal:

A seven-day package to Rio de Janeiro from New York City, including air fare, hotel and transfers, was offered at $599 which was $435 off the regular price. But after receiving notice, club members had only two days to make a decision, and only eight days to show up at the airport.

Before you sign up for this kind of deal-of-a-lifetime, consider that you'll have to pay regular fare from where you live to departure cities — 30-day-in-advance-booking discounts and the like will be long gone. So your best bet is to join a club near your home, or one offering tours from departure points near you.

Last-minute discount travel clubs operate all over the country. But you must find them — your travel agent won't tell you about them, since they don't pay any commissions. Annual membership fees range from $25 to $45. Most of the clubs have newsletters with rundowns on the last-minute deals; some also have telephone hotlines.

Some last-minute travel clubs are listed at the end of this chapter. While, as we said, these discount clubs offer some of the best deals in travel, we have to repeat our earlier warning: if your time isn't flexible, or you have to pay full price for last-minute airfare to some faraway departure city, it may not be such a hot deal, after all. As one travel writer put it, just remember that a bargain isn't really a bargain unless you can use it.

BEWARE OF THOSE 'FREE' TRIPS

Everyone loves a bargain, but be wary whenever anyone offers you a free trip. They're usually trying to sell you something — or worse.

"Good news," says the letter. "You've been computer-selected to receive a free week in the Catskills . . . " Or perhaps it's a "fun-filled week in Florida" or something else like that. Many of those "free" vacations are, not surprisingly, to time-share condos, to golf-course resorts that have lots for sale or to membership campgrounds.

If you're asked to shell out any money — like a "good-faith" deposit, or a "service fee" — find out whether it's refundable and what you have to do to get it back. More than likely, you will have to listen to a sales presentation, and some of those can be pretty intimidating.

Our best advice is to not pay anything at all for a "free" trip — some are out-and-out ripoffs. You get a "free" $1,000 trip to Las Vegas and are asked to put up a $50 "service deposit" — but when you get there, you find you've got one night in a $20 room. Or worse — no reservations at all. Orlando's another popular "free" vacation spot.

If you receive an offer of a free or low-cost travel package, try to find out the real price — chances are, you won't be able to. If you're called on the telephone with such an offer, never give out your credit card number to "guarantee reservations," or for any other reason. If the company wants to send a messenger to swap a travel package for your check or money order, forget it — that's their attempt to avoid postal inspectors.

No matter how alluring those free offers seem, remember that your best bargains in travel come from legitimate travel vendors.

IN SUMMARY:

— Using a good travel agent can save you money.
— Have your destination, your budget and your timing
  planned when you visit a travel agent.

— On major trips, discount travel agents can save you big money — but you have to make most of the arrangements yourself.

— Beware of "free trip" offers.

★ ★ ★
Travel Tool
★ ★ ★

LAST-MINUTE TRAVEL CLUBS

There are hundreds of last-minute travel clubs around the country, most charging small membership fees. Remember that the clubs nearest you are more likely to offer trips departing from your area.

Chicago
Stand-Buys Ltd., 311 W. Superior, Suite 414, Chicago, IL 60610;
☎ toll-free 800/621-5839. Has regional hotlines across the U.S.

Florida
South Florida Cruises, 2005 Cypress Creek Rd., Suite D207, Ft. Lauderdale, FL 33309;
☎ toll-free 800/327-7447. Worldwide Discount Travel Club, 1674 Meridian Ave., Miami Beach, FL 33139;
☎ phone 305/534-2082.

Los Angeles
Spur Of The Moment Cruises, 10780 Jefferson Blvd., Culver City, CA 90230; ☎ toll-free 800/343-1991.

Michigan
Stand-Buys Ltd., P.O. Box 2088, Southfield, MI 48037;
toll-free ☎ 800/621-5839, in Michigan ☎ 800/643-9466.

New England
Last Minute Travel Club, 6A Glenville Ave., Allston, MA 02134;
☎ phone 617/254-5200.
Up'n Go Travel, 10 Mechanic St., Worcester, MA 01608;
☎ phone 508/792-5500.

New York
Moment's Notice
40 E. 49th St., New York, NY 10017;
☎ toll-free 800/253-4321, in New York 212/486-0503.

Northwest
Moment's Notice, 1 Park Place Bldg., Seattle, WA 98101;
☎ phone 206/625-0900. On Call To Travel, P.O. Box 11622, Portland, OR 97211;
☎ phone 503/287-7215.

Philadelphia
Discount Travel International, Ives Bldg., Ste. 205, Norbeth, PA 19151; ☎ toll-free 800/228-6500.

Texas
Vacations To Go, 5901-D Westheimer Rd., Houston, TX 77057;
☎ toll-free 800/624-7338, in Texas 713/974-2121. Has 40 regional telephone hotlines.

Washington, D.C.
Adventures On Call, P.O. Box 18592, Baltimore-Washington International Airport, MD 21240. Encore Travel Card, 4501 Forbes Blvd., Suite. 100, Lanham, MD 20706;
☎ toll-free 800/638-8976.

CHAPTER 4

ARMCHAIR TRAVEL

| How to Cope with the Information Overload |

S it back in your armchair and dream. Put yourself right into gorgeous photos of the Rockies or a Caribbean island; taste from the best restaurants in Paris, the best wines from Burgundy. Check into the boutique hotels of San Francisco. Shop the jade merchants of Hong Kong, or the straw markets of Jamaica. Relax on a sun-splashed Florida beach — or one in Rio.

And do it all before you go. Get the idea?

That's what travel literature will do for you. Read as much of it as you can. Invest the time before you go, and it will save you both time and money once you're there. You'll avoid seeing and doing things that don't really interest you; you'll learn about attractions you didn't know were there.

No matter where you plan to go in this world, you'll have no trouble finding information about it. Indeed, your problem will be information overload. Even if you get only the free stuff, there'll be more literature about your destination than you could possibly absorb.

The British Tourist Authority, for example, has estimated it prints more than 1,000 different brochures for tourists — and there are thousands and thousands more: travel brochures from tour packagers and transportation companies, hundreds of different guidebooks and directories, newsletters, maps, endless articles in travel magazines, coffee-table picture books.

And if you don't like to read, you don't even have to in this electronic age — just slip a travel video into your VCR. How can you possibly miss anything once you get there?

Easy. Those who send you the pretty brochures free-of-charge want to sell you a trip. They don't want you to think about the London fog or the choked ground facilities at Heathrow Airport; those things don't make pretty pictures.

On the other hand, leading guidebook writers, most of whom try to give honest evaluations of everything from restaurants to the genealogy of the Loch Ness Monster, don't seem to agree on much of anything. The hotel described in one guidebook as having "old-world charm" is called "cramped and crowded, without private baths" in another.

Just who do you believe, anyhow? The best answer is your own instincts.

HOW TO READ THE TRAVEL BROCHURES

Travel brochures can be useful in helping you select what kind of trip to take and where to go. And don't let the word "brochure" fool you — many of these are big printed catalogs, with hundreds of pages and splashy color photos.

Your travel agent will load you down with brochures from airlines, tour packagers, resorts and cruiselines. Or if you're planning the trip by yourself, you can write for a mountain of brochures just from ads in your Sunday paper or travel magazine.

Even if you've already selected your destination, travel brochures can play a large part in determining how you get there, and how well you read them will determine whether you'll enjoy your journey. You will get more pretty pictures and less information per pound from these brochures than from any other kind of travel publication. Remember that the brochures — except for the small print on the back pages — are sales tools. Those who create the brochures are paid to make the tours sound good, and they'll use every creative trick of words and graphics to do that.

Nevertheless, mature travelers who pay attention to the words as well as the pictures can glean a lot of information from brochures, and be able to compare one tour against another.

Test the words — Your "airy" room may turn out to be lacking air-conditioning. "First class" rooms in one country may be a lot classier than in another country, even though there are standard definitions (see Chapter 5, Lodging). Find out what those terms mean for the particular tour you're interested in. "Near golf courses" usually means you've got to take a taxi to get there. Does "deluxe motorcoach" mean there's a bathroom on the bus? And ask whether the tour is "fully escorted" or whether you're on your own to get from plane to hotel or other places. Don't assume anything.

How long is the trip? — A "one-week" trip can be six nights and seven days — two of which you'll spend getting there and back. If you're planning a trip abroad, remember that recovering from jet lag could steal another day from your schedule. Some cruiselines call "a three-day trip" one that departs at 4:30 p.m. Friday and returns at 8 a.m. Monday.

Who pays? — "Golf available," even at a golf-course resort, means you'll pay extra to play. "Optional sightseeing" means it's not included in the tour price—there's an extra charge whenever the brochure uses the letter "O," for "optional." And find out whether the tour price includes transfers — that is, the cost of getting from the airport to your hotel, tips and the like.

How many meals? — One brochure says, "Some meals are skipped so you can dine out, have a light snack or spend time doing something else." That's another way of saying, "All meals are not included." Ask how many are included in the tour price whether you can eat anything on the menu and who does the tipping.

A free pamphlet, *Let's Talk Travel*, explains some expressions, abbreviations and frequently used travel terms that will help you evaluate the travel brochures. Send a stamped, addressed envelope to the Institute of Certified Travel Agents, 148 Linden St., P.O. Box 56, Wellesley, MA 02181.

A final clue for seniors in evaluating cruises and tours depicted in the brochures is the pictures. People who create brochures are very careful about the mood they create through pictures. Do the pictures show young people, beer cans in hand, having wild fun? Or do they show older folks sipping wine and chatting by the pool?

Through the photos, they are trying to address their preferred audiences — youngsters on a budget to mature travelers on an upscale cruise.

Try to stay tuned in to all the clues in a brochure.

OTHER FREE STUFF

After you've picked your destination or route, figure out what there is to see and do there. This is where the free literature helps.

Whether you're visiting the Garlic Festival in Gilroy, Calif., or the Running of the Bulls in Pamplona, Spain, write the local tourism authority or chamber of commerce for all the free literature you can get. Every place that's tourist-oriented has an organization that dispenses such information.

Addresses and phone numbers of state tourism agencies, and those of selected countries, are at the end of this chapter.

In your letter, state your itinerary and the time of year you'll be there — you'll get a far different package, for example, from the State of Minnesota for a summer visit than for a winter one. Ask for maps, walking tours, guidebooks, hotel lists, restaurants, lists of attractions, calendars of events and anything else they can send — let them know you're serious.

If you're planning an extended trip — say, a drive across the U.S. or a motorcoach trip to several destinations — don't forget to write every place you'll go through. If you're headed for the Rockies, you might be surprised at some of the things you can visit on your overnight stays in Missouri and Kansas.

☎ ☎ ☎
USING TOLL-FREE NUMBERS

Instead of writing, you can get lots of the information you need for your budget planning quicker by using toll-free 800 numbers. Every hotel and motel chain has one that feeds into a central reservation switchboard where you can get quotes on rates and facilities for any member of the chain. Later you can use these same toll-free numbers to price-shop for a room where you've decided to visit, and to make reservations.

When you research this way, remember that central switchboards quote only published rates and company-wide deals, not specials that local units may not have told them about. A wine country Ramada Inn was recently offering seniors 40 percent discounts, while Ramada central reservation was quoting only the standard 25 percent off regular rates. When you arrive at the inn, be sure to ask for any special promotional rates better than the one you were quoted.

Cruiselines and tour operators also have toll-free numbers that you can call for prices and free brochures. Many of them are in this book; many of them are advertised in your Sunday newspaper travel section.

If you call toll-free 800 numbers frequently, it will save time if you subscribe to the AT&T Toll-Free 800 Consumer Directory for less than $10 a year. Write AT&T 800 Directory, P.O. Box 44068, Jacksonville, FL 32232-4068 for an order form, or call 800/426-8686.

You can also get any toll free number from an information operator — dial 800/555-1212.

TRAVEL MAGAZINES

People who take travel seriously subscribe to one or more of the leading travel magazines: *Travel & Leisure*, *Travel-Holiday*, *Conde' Nast's Traveler* or the *National Geographic Traveler*. And they never throw away an issue.

Here's where you'll learn the real fun of discovery.

Sitting at home, we were trying to get a line on a few good, affordable restaurants in Burgundy and Paris — places we had never been. Sure enough, in our stack of *T&Ls* was a recent article on six undiscovered restaurants in Paris, and an older article on eating in the French wine country. We picked out three restaurants in Paris and a few in Burgundy and wrote them down. None of these restaurants was listed in the guidebook we'd decided to use, though the book had always led us to restaurants we liked.

Between those in the guidebook and those in the magazine, we never had a bad meal in France.

The payoff came one night at a mom-and-pop restaurant in Paris featuring country-French cuisine, a restaurant *T&L* thought should rate right up there with Maxim's. Well, it did. Not only that, but because the magazine had printed the proprietor's photo, we were able to greet him by name in our broken French. The fact that his fame had suddenly traveled to far-off America was too much. His wife wept, and the owner-chef, we're sure, made us the finest meal he'd ever worked on. Thanks, *T&L*.

The point is that if you want to explore off-the-beaten-path on your next trip — whether it's abroad or in this country — articles in these mainstream travel magazines will lead you to the hidden surprises that make travel so much fun — places you won't find in the standard guidebooks. And the information will be about as fresh as you can get it.

When you get ready to search for articles for trip planning, you don't even have to go through the magazines one-by-one. They're travelers' helpers — many of these magazines are indexed on the spine. Just look along the spines to find the places you're interested in.

If you don't subscribe, most public libraries carry at least one or two of these four magazines.

GUIDEBOOKS

A good guidebook should tell you everything you need to know about your destination that will make your trip more enjoyable. It's the one book you should carry along on your trip.

Don't use a guidebook to choose your destination — you don't want to get bogged down in trolley schedules, foreign phrases, best hotels, tipping practices and the like in that early stage of planning. Rather, use a guidebook to help you get around once you arrive.

Most travel guides are part of a prominent series: Fodor's, Fielding's, Frommer's and so on. Though these are the old reliables, occasionally you'll find an individual guide to a particular area that stands head-and-shoulders above any of the standard series.

There are well over 1,000 travel guidebooks available today, and even more directories. How do you choose one?

You can ask your travel agent, who likely has read more guides than anybody. You can ask a friend, who's actually tested a guidebook or two on trips. Or you can ask a bookseller.

"People often ask my advice about travel books because the choice is so overwhelming," says the manager of a major bookstore in California. "I make suggestions on the basis of popularity and customer comments." On sales, she means — as good a test as any.

The best way to pick a guidebook is the personal test: Take one along on your next trip, and if it doesn't lead you astray and if it gives you information that makes your trip more enjoyable, that's the series to stick with.

The good guidebooks are updated frequently, which makes them more expensive. Never rely on a travel guidebook more than two years old — those updated yearly are even more reliable. Look for the copyright date inside the cover.

Yearly updates cost a publisher more, which increases the price of the guide. Choose a guidebook for its content — not its price. A cheap guide can cost you more money with bad advice and lost opportunities than you'd ever believe.

The editor's intent and personal tastes also account for much of the difference in guidebooks. Guidebook Editor Arthur Frommer once said: "Our authors personally enjoy staying at non-standard, less pretentious places, and our tour books are for readers who enjoy the same." Which gives Frommer guides appeal to the traveler on a budget. Stephen Birnbaum's guides, on the other hand, take an upscale approach in comments and ratings.

Many guides, like AAA's and Michelin's, rate restaurants and inns. Other guides don't even mention them. If you're not an eater, and a bed to you is just a place to stop between sightseeing trips, don't worry about the ratings — get a guidebook that describes the sights and gives insights on other attractions you are interested in. Perhaps you'd prefer a guidebook that rates castles or beaches, or gives you information on local customs, rather than the best places to sightsee.

The only way to pick a guidebook initially is to spend some time in a travel bookstore, or one of the big chains, browsing the shelves. Read some passages to find out if the guide offers the kind of information you want. And if you've got a favorite restaurant, hotel or attraction from some previous trip elsewhere, see if you agree on how a sister guidebook rates it.

✔✔✔

Here are some of the leading travel guide series. Except for AAA's, all are available in bookstores:

AAA Tour Books — What to see and where to stay when traveling by auto in the U.S., Canada, Mexico or Europe. Has city maps. Over the years, we've found AAA's ratings of hotels and restaurants to be very accurate. AAA also puts out a series of *Campbooks*, which rate campgrounds for RVers and tenters. Free to AAA members; not available to others. If you're not a member, *Mobil Guides* (below) are good substitutes.

American Express — Pocket-size guides to U.S. and Europe are packed with maps, information on sights, hotels, restaurants, thanks to space-saving symbols used and small print. Writing is lively and informative. A companion book, *American Express International Traveler's Pocket Dictionary and Phrase Book*, comes in four editions: French, German, Italian and Spanish.

Berlitz Travel Guides— How to get around in individual cities. Small and convenient to carry. Lots of helpful foreign phrases.

Birnbaum Guides--North and South American and European guides take an upscale approach to sightseeing, shopping, lodgings and dining.

Fielding Travel Guides — Cover whole continents, and contain a toll-free number for updates and any personal travel questions. Tough, witty evaluations appeal to upscale travelers.

Fodor Guides — The series, which covers the globe, aims for a middle-of-the road audience in terms of finances and experience.

The Arthur Frommer Guides: The *Dollar Wise Guides* — Emphasize value, though listings include all price ranges. Titles range from all of Europe to individual European countries and Hawaii.

The Michelin Guides — The green books offer detailed descriptions of all the sights in a country or major city. Be sure you select the guide written in English. The famous *Michelin Red Books* are still the leading guides that rate restaurants and lodging places — and they're small enough to carry with you when you dine.

Mobil Travel Guides--Same kind of information as AAA books, except just for the United States and Canada. Available in bookstores. We use Mobil and AAA guides to plan advance reservations at new destinations and along the way. Both update their information yearly.

TRAVEL DIRECTORIES

There are directories for almost any subject you can think of, anywhere in the world — lists of museums in Oklahoma, cathedrals in Germany, country inns in Scotland, chateaux in Picardy, campgrounds in America, B&Bs for almost every state, and so on.

Directories usually give address and phone number, description and other pertinent information for whatever they're listing. Many, like directories of hotels and restaurants, are put out by the hotel and restaurant companies. Some are sponsored by trade groups, like chambers of commerce and area restaurant associations, and list only their members — good and bad. A directory that's sponsored, that has paid listings, or one that doesn't cost you any money is likely to be incomplete and could even lead you astray.

There are directories you can buy, however, that are useful as guides for making advance reservations, planning itineraries and the like.

TRAVEL BOOKS

Author James Michener, when he was 81, said before you travel someplace, read a book about it:

"Any of the great travel books is as good as any fiction."

Michener's favorites included *A Confederacy of Dunces* (Grove Press, $4.50) by John Kennedy Toole for the flavor of life in New Orleans; *The Milagro Beanfield War* (Ballantine, $4.95) by John Nichols for a look at Mexican-American life in the Southwest; and *Playing God in Yellowstone* (Harcourt Brace Jovanovich, $10.95) by Alston Chase for a description of the National Park Service's work in Yellowstone.

He could have included some of his own books, like *South Pacific, Hawaii* and *Centennial* for stimulating interest in travel, as well. Steinbeck, Hemingway and even Louis L'Amour wrote classic books that stimulated people to travel to the places described.

Some of the best fiction, indeed, lives forever. That can't be said, however, of most travel books. They go out-of-date too quickly. Unlike guidebooks, general books on travel, whether they tell readers how to travel or where to travel, are rarely updated. And the great little restaurants and hideaway shops that were there last year may not be there this year

One of the least useful kinds of travel books we've found are those full of travel discounts for seniors. One recently came across our desk with the pretentious title *Unbelievably Good Deals & Great Adventures That You Absolutely Can't Get Unless You're Over 50*. All the information was old — things that you probably already knew — and many of the deals simply were no longer offered by the time we got our review copy.

Paige Palmer's *Senior Citizen's Guides to Budget Travel* in the U.S., Canada and Europe, as well-researched as they are, suffer from the same thing.

The problem any author labors under is the enormous lead time required to get a book into print. And deals for seniors are a moving target — they come and go too quickly to be a proper topic for a full book. That's why people read newsletters.

Select a book to catch the flavor of your destination, its history, its customs. But don't believe what you read about special deals or special places, unless the book is less than two years old.

SOME UNIQUE DIRECTORY/BOOKS

Books we especially like, whether to help plan a trip or to tell us what to find when we get there, are Prentice Hall's *Places Rated* series and John Howells' *Retirement Choices* (Gateway Books).

There are a *Places Rated Almanac, Sports Places Rated, Vacation Places Rated and Retirement Places Rated*. The last two are especially good for travel planning.

It's not that we believe in their final ratings (who wants to retire in Iowa City, Iowa, just because they've got lots of doctors and a good bus system?). It's the descriptions of places that we find valuable — mountains of statistics ranging from golf holes per capita to the number of starred restaurants, as well as conventional descriptions of what there is to see and do.

Even the ratings make good conversation ("Say, did you know Traverse City, Mich., is one of the top sports towns in America?" "Naw — tell that to the Dodgers." "Well, that's what it says . . .) — or even some good fistfights.

TRAVEL NEWSLETTERS

Travel newsletters fill the information cracks that books and magazines can't. They're the only really fresh source of information that's available regularly.

While the information in a book may be a year old before it gets to print, the newsletter in your mailbox may have news less than a week old. Even magazine lead times are two to six months, and that's too long to be useful for a frequent traveler. Deals and trips for 49ers-plus are a moving target. They come and go quickly.

If you're a frequent traveler, taking two or more trips a year, subscribe to a good newsletter in an area that interests you. It's the only way to take advantage of attractive offerings when they appear.

There are as many as 70 newsletters about travel. They start up and fold at an alarming rate, and any comprehensive listing would be out-of-date almost instantly. Many newsletters concentrate on tiny parts of the world: (¡Mexico West!, or The Las Vegas Connection). Some are just for upscale travelers, and tell of expensive little hideaways the average traveler never sees (The Privileged Traveler); others cover dude ranching, B&Bs, freighter travel and all kinds of other specialties. One even covers travel for seniors (The Mature Traveler, see below).

To survey the newsletter field and find one that interests you, find a copy of Oxbridge Directory of Newsletters (15,000 listings) or Gale's Newsletter Directory (10,000 listings) at your public library. All the information you need to subscribe will be there.

Here are some newsletters mature travelers will find particularly useful:

Around and About Travel — For the physically challenged traveler, has reports from readers, accessibility updates, listings of tours and publications. Bimonthly. $20/year. 931 Shoreline Dr., San Mateo, CA 94404, ☎ 415/573-7998.

Consumer Reports Travel Letter — Offspring of Consumer Reports magazine, and just as thorough in its analyses. Tedious reading sometimes, but lots of details like fare comparisons, best deals in everything from hotel rooms to rental cars. Stresses consumer affairs, but there are some destination stories. Monthly. $37/year. Box 53629, Boulder, CO 80322-3629. ☎ Phone toll-free 800/525-0643.

Freighter Travel News--Detailed accounts of freighter travel trips, listings of worldwide offerings. $18/year. Published monthly by Freighter Travel Club of America, P.O. Box 12693, Salem, OR 97309.

International Travel News--Big tabloid full of punchy travel reports from readers, currency rates, hotel and restaurant reviews, reader commentary, travel trivia. Monthly. $14/year. 2120 28th St., Sacramento, CA 95818. ☎ 916/457-3643.

The Mature Traveler — Published by the authors of this book, this is the only newsletter specifically for 49ers-plus. Packed with current bargains for seniors, trips for seniors; roundups on hotel deals, airfare deals, singles travel clubs, cruises; reports on destinations for mature travelers; travel-partner-wanted ads. Monthly. $21.97/year. P.O. Box 50820, Reno, *NV 89513.*

Travel Smart — Breezy letter reveals inside deals; analyses of things like frequent-flyer programs, ski resorts; strong on adventure travel. Monthly. $37/year. 40 Beechdale Rd., Dobbs Ferry, NY 10522. Phone toll-free ☎ 800/327-3633.

TRAVEL VIDEOS

Remember the glorious travelogues we used to see as short subjects at the movies? Well, they're still around. Except now they're on video cassettes, and you can watch them in your own home.

Michael Kong, publisher of the *Travel Video Directory*, estimates there are more than 300 travel videos available today. There are 25 on Hawaii, alone.

These travelogues made a comeback in the early 1980s, mostly so travel agents could watch them and learn more about the trips they were selling. Now travel agents share them with clients, either showing them in the office or lending them.

You can also buy travelogues for your own library, at $5 to $40. They range in length from 8 to 90 minutes — the longer they are, the more you're likely to learn.

But the caveat is the same as for the printed free stuff — remember that the people who make those videos are trying to get you to come there; they are painting a pretty picture. And no video can cram into even 90 minutes the information you'll get from a good guidebook.

Here are some places to get lists of travel videos for sale:

American Express Tapes, c/o Preview Media, 1160 Berry St., Suite 100, San Francisco, CA 94111. ☎ toll-free 800/992-8439. 15 titles.

Chronicle Videocassettes, P.O. Box 708, Northbrook, IL 60065. ☎ Phone toll-free 800/445-3800. 15 titles.

Vacations on Video, 1309 E. Northern, Phoenix, AZ 85020. ☎ 602/840-2732. 300 titles.

International Adventure Video, 680 Waverly St., Palo Alto, CA 94301. ☎ 415/321-9943. 108 titles.

For the *Travel Video Directory*, send $17.50 to Travel Video Association, 2 Mott St., New York, NY 10013. ☎ 212/580-3366.

TRAVEL BOOKSTORES

If you're a travel junkie, you're blessed if you live near a large city where one of the two dozen or more travel specialty bookstores is located. You can spend hours in one, browsing among the maps and guidebooks and magazines and travel trinkets they sell. It's a place where you have a chance to open the guidebooks and compare entries, to find out without buying which one fits your style of travel

Even if there's not a travel bookstore in your area, major book dealers like B. Dalton and Waldenbooks have large travel sections, and if they don't carry a book you read about here, they'll usually be able to order it for you.

Some travel bookstores do a big mail-order business, and put out catalogs for those who can't come in. You'll find that just browsing through the titles can set your travel juices coursing. Free catalogs of travel books are available from:

Book Passage, 51 Tamal Vista Blvd., Corte Madera, CA 94925, near San Francisco. ☎ toll-free 800/321-9785.

The Complete Traveller, 199 Madison Ave., New York, NY 10016. ☎ 212/685-9007.

Forsyth Travel Library, 9154 W. 57th St., P.O. Box 2975, Shawnee Mission, KS 66201, in a suburb of Kansas City. ☎ Call toll-free 800/367-7984.

Phileas Fogg's Books and Maps, 87 Stanford Shopping Center, Palo Alto, CA 94304. ☎ Toll-free 800/533-3644 (in California 800/233-3644).

Travel Books Unlimited, 4931 Cordell Ave., Bethesda, MD 20814.

Wayfarer Books, P.O. Box 1121, Davenport, IA 52805.

Wide World Bookshop, 401 N.E. 45th St., Seattle, WA 98105.

IN SUMMARY:

— Write tourist authorities for all the free information you can get.
— Read the travel brochures skeptically for code words and other clues.
— Subscribe to a good travel magazine.
— Regularly read a travel newsletter in a field that interests you.
— Take along a guidebook you agree with.

★ ★ ★
Travel Tool
★ ★ ★

WHERE TO GET FREE TRAVEL INFORMATION IN THE U.S.

Here's where to write or phone the states for free literature. State tourism agencies can put you in touch with individual city or area agencies.

Alabama Bureau of Tourism & Travel
532 S. Perry St.
Montgomery, AL 36104
☎ 800/633-5761

Alaska Division of Tourism
P.O. Box E
Juneau, AK 99811
☎ 907/465-2010

Arizona Office of Tourism
1480 Bethany Home Rd., Suite 180
Phoenix, AZ 85014
☎ 602/255-4764

Arkansas Tourism Office
1 Capitol Mall, Dept. 7701
Little Rock, AR 72201
☎ 800/643-8383

California Office of Tourism
1121 L St., Suite 10
Sacramento, CA 95814
☎ 916/322-2881

Colorado Tourism Board
1625 Broadway, Suite 1700
Denver, CO 80202
☎ 800/433-2656

Connecticut Tourism Promotion Service
Department of Economic Development
210 Washington St., Rm. 900
Hartford, CT 06106
☎ 800/243-1685

Delaware Tourism Office
99 Kings Highway
P.O. Box 1401
Dover, DE 19903
☎ 800/441-8846

D.C. Convention & Visitors Assn.
1575 Eye St. NW, Suite 250
Washington, DC 20005
☎ 202/789-7000

Florida Division of Tourism
126 Van Buren St.
Tallahassee, FL 32309-2000
☎ 904/487-1462

Georgia Department of Industry & Trade
P.O. Box 1776
Atlanta, GA 30301
☎ 404/656-3590

Hawaii Visitors Bureau
P.O. Box 8527
Honolulu, HI 96815
☎ 808/923-1811

Idaho Travel Council
Statehouse, Dept. C
Boise, ID 83720
☎ 800/635-7820

Illinois Tourist Information Center
310 S. Michigan Ave., Suite 108
Chicago, IL 60604
☎ 800/232-0121

Indiana Dept. of Commerce
Tourism Division
1 North Capitol, Suite 700
Indianapolis, IN 46204
☎ 317/232-8860

Iowa Department of Economic Development
Bureau of Visitors and Tourism
200 E. Grand P.O. Box 6127
Des Moines, IA 50309
☎ 515/281-3100

Kansas Tourism & Travel Division
Department of Economic Development
400 W. Eighth St., 5th Fl.
Topeka, KS 66603
☎ 913/296-2009

Kentucky Department of Travel & Development
2200 Capital Plaza Tower
Frankfort, KY 40601
☎ 800/225-8747

Louisiana Office of Tourism
P.O. Box 94291
Baton Rouge, LA 70804-9291
☎ 800/334-8626

Maine Division of Tourism
97 Winthrop St.
Hallowell, ME 04347-2300
☎ 800/533-9595

Maryland Office of Tourist Development
45 Calvert St.
Annapolis, MD 21401
☎ 800/331-1750, Op. 250

Massachusetts Office of Travel & Tourism
100 Cambridge St.
Boston, MA 02202
☎ 800/624-6277

Michigan Travel Bureau
Department of Commerce
P.O. Box 30226
Lansing, MI 48909
☎ 800/543-2937

Minnesota Office of Tourism
375 Jackson St.
St. Paul, MN 55101
☎ 800/328-1461

Mississippi Division of Tourism
Department of Economic Development
P.O. Box 22825
Jackson, MS 39205
☎ 800/647-2290

Missouri Division of Tourism
P.O. Box 1055
Jefferson City, MO 65102
☎ 314/751-4133

Travel Montana
Room 835
Deerlodge, MT 59722
☎ 800/541-1447

Nebraska Division of Travel & Tourism
P.O. Box 94666, Rm. 88937
Lincoln, NE 68509
☎ 800/228-4307

Nevada Commission on Tourism
Capitol Complex
Carson City, NV 89710
☎ 800/638-2328

New Hampshire Office of Vacation Travel
P.O. Box 856
Concord, NH 03301
☎ 603/271-2665

New Jersey Division of Travel & Tourism
20 W. State St.
Trenton, NJ 08625
☎ 800/537-7397

New Mexico
Tourism & Travel Division
Joseph M. Montoya Bldg.
1100 St. Francis Dr., Rm. 777
Santa Fe, NM 87503
☎ 800/545-2040

New York State Commerce Department
1 Commerce Plaza
Albany, NY 12245
☎ 800/225-5697 (Eastern states only)
☎ 518/474-4116

North Carolina Travel & Tourism Division
Department of Commerce
430 N. Salisbury St.
Raleigh, NC 27611
☎ 800/847-4862

North Dakota Tourism Promotion
Liberty Memorial Bldg., Rm. 250
Capitol Grounds
Bismarck, ND 58505
☎ 800/437-2077

Ohio Department of Travel & Tourism
P.O. Box 1001
Columbus, OH 43266
☎ 800/282-5393

Oklahoma Tourism & Recreation Department
Marketing Services Division
500 Will Rogers Bldg.
Oklahoma City, OK 73105
☎ 800/652-6552

Oregon Tourism Division
Oregon Economic Development
595 Cottage St., N.E.
Salem, OR 97310
☎ 800/547-7842

Pennsylvania Bureau of Travel Development
416 Forum Bldg., Dept. PR901
Harrisburg, PA 17120
☎ 800/847-4072

Puerto Rico Tourism Development Co.
P.O. Box 025268, Dept. H
Miami, FL 33102-5268
☎ 800/233-6530

Rhode Island Department of Economic Development
Tourism Department
7 Jackson Walkway
Providence, RI 02903
☎ 800/556-2484 (Eastern states only)
☎ 401/277-2601

South Carolina Division of Tourism
P.O. Box 71, Rm. 902
Columbia, SC 29202
☎ 803/734-0122

South Dakota Division of Tourism
Capitol Lake Plaza
711 Wells Ave.
Pierre, SD 57501
☎ 800/843-8000

Tennessee Department of Tourism Development
P.O. Box 23170
Nashville, TN 37202
☎ 615/741-2158

Texas Tourist Development Agency
P.O. Box 12008
Austin, TX 78711
☎ 512/462-9191

Utah Travel Council
Council Hall, Capitol Hill
Salt Lake City, UT 84114
☎ 801/533-5681

Vermont Travel Division
134 State St.
Montpelier, VT 05602
☎ 802/828-3236

Virgin Islands Division of Tourism
P.O. Box 6400
Charlotte Amalie, St. Thomas, USVI 00801
☎ 800/372-8784

Virginia Division of Tourism
202 N. Ninth St., Suite 500
Richmond, VA 23219
☎ 804/786-2051

Washington State Tourism Development Division
General Administration Bldg. AX-13
Olympia, WA 98504-0613
☎ 800/544-1800

West Virginia Department of Commerce
Marketing/Tourism Division
Charleston, WV 25305
☎ 800/225-5982

Wisconsin Division of Tourism Development
Box 7606 Madison, WI 53707
☎ 800/432-8747

Wyoming Travel Commission
I-25 at College Drive
Cheyenne, WY 82002-0660
☎ 307/777-7777

Travel Tool
★ ★ ★

WHERE TO GET FREE FOREIGN TRAVEL INFORMATION

Here's where to write for literature for your trip abroad:

Arab Information Center
1100 17th St. N.W., Suite 602
Washington, DC 20036
☎ 202/265-3210
(Handles requests for Algeria, Iraq, Jordan, Kuwait, Lebanon, Libya, Mauritania, Morocco, North Yemen, Oman, Qatar, Saudi Arabia, Somalia, Sudan, Syria, Tunisia, United Arab Emirates, Yemen- -Offices also in Chicago, N.Y., Dallas)

Argentine Republic Embassy
1600 New Hampshire Ave., N.W.
Washington, DC 20009
☎ 202/939-6400

Aruba Tourism Authority
521 Fifth Avenue, 12th Floor
New York, NY 10175
☎ 212/246-3030

Austrian National Tourist Office
489 Fifth Ave.
New York, NY 10117
☎ 212/687-6300
(Offices also in Chicago, L.A.)

Australian Tourist Commission
2121 Avenue of the Stars
Los Angeles, CA 90067
☎ 213/552-1988
(Offices also in N.Y., Chicago)

Bahamas Islands Tourist Office
255 Alhambra Circle
Coral Gables, FL 33134
☎ 800/327-7678
(Offices also in other major U.S. and Canadian cities)

Belgian Tourist Office
745 Fifth Ave.

New York, NY 10151
☎ 212/758-8130
(Office also in Montreal)

Bermuda Department of Tourism
630 Fifth Ave.
New York, NY 10111
☎ 212/397-7700
(Offices also in Atlanta, Chicago, Boston, Toronto)

Brazilian Tourism Foundation
551 Fifth Ave., Rm. 519
New York, NY 10176
☎ 212/286-9600

British Tourist Authority
40 W. 57th St.
New York, NY 10019
☎ 212/581-4700
(England, Scotland, Wales, Northern Ireland — Offices also in Chicago, Dallas, L.A., Toronto, Vancouver)

Canada — Contact the following provincial tourist offices:

Travel Alberta
P.O. Box 2500
Edmonton, Alta., Canada T5J 2Z4
☎ 800/661-8888

Tourism B.C.
562 Burrard St.
Vancouver, B.C. Canada V6C 2J6
☎ 800/663-6000

Travel Manitoba
Dept. 5020, Legislative Bldg.
Winnipeg, Man., Canada R3C 0V8
☎ 800/665-0040

Tourism New Brunswick
P.O. Box 12345
Fredericton, N.B, Canada E3B 5C3
☎ 800/561-0123

Newfoundland Tourism Branch
Department of Development
Box 2016
St. John's, Newfoundland, Canada A1C 5R8
☎ 800/563-6353

Northwest Territories Travel Arctic
Yellowknife
Northwest Territories, Canada X1A 2L9
☎ 800/661-0788

Nova Scotia Tourist Information Office
129 Commerical St.Portland, ME 04101
☎ 800/341-6096

Ontario Ministry of Tourism
77 Bloor St. W.
Toronto, Ont., Canada M7A 2R9
☎ 800/268-3735

Prince Edward Island
Department of Tourism
P.O. Box 940
Charlottetown
Prince Edward Island, Canada C1A 7M5
☎ 902/368-4444

Tourisme Quebec
Stock Exchange
800 Place, No. 260 B.P. 125
Montreal, P.Q. Canada H4Z1C3
☎ 514/873-2015

Tourism Saskatchewan
2103 11th Ave.
Regina, Sask., Canada S4P 3V7
☎ 800/667-7191

Tourism Yukon
P.O. Box 2703
Whitehorse, Yukon, Canada Y1A 2C6
☎ 403/667-5430

Caribbean Tourism Association
20 E. 46th St.
New York, NY 10017
☎ 212/682-0435

(For information on all Caribbean islands, plus Venezuela, Surinam, Panama, Curaçao, Costa Rica)

China
The People's Republic has no U.S. tourism offices yet, but see Hong Kong listing.

Egyptian Government Tourist Office
523 Geary St., Suite 303
San Francisco, CA 94102

French Government Tourist Office
610 Fifth Ave.
New York, NY 10020
☎ 212/757-1125
(Offices also in Chicago, Dallas, L.A., San Francisco, Montreal, Toronto)

German National Tourist Office
747 Third Ave.
New York, NY 10017
☎ 212/308-3300

Greek National Tourist Organization
645 Fifth Ave.
New York, NY 10022
☎ 212/421-5777
(Offices also in Chicago, L.A., Montreal, Toronto)

Hong Kong Tourist Assn.
160 Sansome St.
San Francisco, CA 94104
☎ 415/989-5005
(Also handles queries for People's Republic of China — Offices also in other major U.S. cities)

India Tourist Office
30 Rockefeller Plaza
New York, NY 10112
☎ 212/586-4901
(Offices also in other U.S. and Canadian cities)

Indonesian Tourist Promotion Bd.
323 Geary St.
San Francisco, CA 94102
☎ 415/981-3585

Irish Tourist Board
757 Third Ave.
New York, NY 10017
☎ 212/418-0800
(Offices also in San Francisco, L.A., Toronto)

Israel Government Tourist Office
350 Fifth Ave.
New York, NY 10018
☎ 212/560-0650
(Offices also in L.A., Atlanta, Chicago, Toronto)

Italian Government Travel Office
630 Fifth Ave.
New York, NY 10111
☎ 212/245-4822
(Offices also in Chicago, San Francisco, Dallas, Montreal)

Jamaica Tourist Board
1320 S. Dixie Hwy.
Coral Gables, FL 33146
☎ 305/665-0557
(Offices also in L.A., Chicago, N.Y., Toronto)

Japan National Tourist Organization
630 Fifth Ave., Suite 2101
New York, NY 10111
☎ 212/757-5460
(Offices also in L.A., San Francisco, Chicago, Dallas, Toronto)

Kenya Tourist Office
424 Madison Ave.
New York, N.Y. 10017
☎ 212/486-1300
(Office also in Beverly Hills, Washington)

Korean National Tourism Corp.
460 Park Ave.
New York, NY 10022
☎ 212/688-7543
(Offices also in L.A., Honolulu, Chicago, Seattle)

Luxembourg National Tourist Office
801 Second Ave.
New York, NY 10017
☎ 212/751-9650

Malaysian Tourist Information Center
818 W. Seventh St.
Los Angeles, CA 90017
☎ 213/689-9702

Mexican National Tourist Council
405 Park Ave., Suite 1002
New York, NY 10022
☎ 800/331-1100
(Offices in many other major U.S. and Canadian cities)

Middle East
(See Arab Information Center)

Monaco Government Tourist Bureau
845 Third Ave.
New York, NY 10022
☎ 212/759-5227

Netherlands Board of Tourism
355 Lexington Ave.
New York, NY 10017
☎ 212/370-7360
(Offices also in Chicago, San Francisco)

New Zealand Government Tourist Office
One Maritime Plaza, Suite 970
San Francisco, CA 94111
☎ 415/788-7404
(Offices also in L.A., N.Y., Toronto)

Pacific Asia Travel Association
One Montgomery St.
Telesis Tower, Suite 1750
San Francisco, CA 94104
☎ 415/986-4646
(Provides information for many Pacific-area destinations, including major island destinations, Australia, Hong Kong, Indonesia, Macau, Nepal, Hawaii, Japan, Malaysia, Philippines, Tahiti, Taiwan, Sri Lanka, Singapore, Papua New Guinea, Pakistan, Thailand, USSR.)

Portuguese National Tourist Office
590 Fifth Ave.
New York, NY 10036
☎ 212/354-4403
(Offices also in Toronto, Montreal)

Scandinavian Tourist Board
655 Third Ave.
New York, NY 10017
☎ 212/949-2333
(Representing Denmark, Finland, Iceland, Norway, Sweden)

Singapore Tourist Promotion Board
8484 Wilshire Blvd., Suite 510
Beverly Hills, CA 90211
☎ 213/852-1901
(Office also in N.Y.)

South Africa Tourist Corp.
747 Third Ave.
New York, NY 10173
☎ 212/838-8841
(Offices also in L.A.)

Spanish National Tourist Office
665 Fifth Ave.
New York, NY 10022
☎ 212/759-8822
(Offices also in San Francisco, Chicago, Houston, Toronto, St. Augustine, Fla.)

Swiss National Tourist Office
608 Fifth Ave.
New York, NY 10020
☎ 212/757-5944
(Offices also in San Francisco, Toronto, Montreal

Taiwan Visitors Association
One World Trade Center, Suite 8855
New York, NY 10048
☎ 212/466-0691
(Offices also in San Francisco, Chicago)

Thailand Tourism Authority
5 World Trade Center
New York, NY 10048
☎ 212/432-0433
(Office also in L.A.)

Turkish Tourism & Information Office
821 United Nations Plaza
New York, NY 10017
☎ 212/687-2194

U.S.S.R. Company for Foreign Travel (Intourist)
630 Fifth Ave.
New York, NY 10111
☎ 212/757-3884
(Office also in Montreal)

Venezuela Government Tourist Bureau
450 Park Ave.
New York, NY 10022
☎ 212/355-1101

Yugoslav National Tourist Office
630 Fifth Ave.
New York, NY 10111
☎ 212/757-2801

NOTES

CHAPTER 5

LODGING

Wherever You Go, Ask for the Discount

No matter where you travel in the United States, Canada or Mexico, never pay the full rate for a room. Ask for the senior-citizen discount, even if one isn't posted. Most major chains, as well as independents, recognize seniors as a group to be courted, and give discounts accordingly — some up to 50 percent. The only exception may be classy independent hotels catering to business travelers.

The story is different overseas, where discounts for mature travelers are less common. But often, you get deep discounts on lodgings there, anyhow, as part of your tour package.

And nowadays there is a wide range of other choices to add adventure to your trip or cut your lodging costs: paradors in Spain, castles in France, B&Bs everywhere, house exchanges, hosted holidays, vacation apartments and more. You can stay in a tepee in Oregon (Kah-Nee-Ta Resort — no senior discount) or save up to $2,000 sleeping in a camper in Europe.

HOW TO PICK AN INN

We were stopping just overnight in London, on the way to somewhere else. Our itinerary, made out by the travel agent, simply said "Cadogan Hotel" and gave the address in the Knightsbridge district. "You'll enjoy this place," the travel agent said. "I've stayed there."

Actually, we only wanted a clean hotel where we could throw off jet lag before our trip the next day. And, surely, it was that.

75

Our cab pulled up in front of a tiny Victorian building, pinched-in between some others that looked identical. Across the street was a park, and three blocks away was a typical workingman's pub, where we had lunch. It was a long walk to Piccadilly, but the Piccadilly bus went right by, which we appreciated.

What made the Cadogan special was that it was Lillie Langtry's hotel — the place she favored for her secret meetings with Edward, Prince of Wales, future king of England. The place where Oscar Wilde wrote sonnets and essays, the place where James Whistler drank. And there were photos and memorabilia all over the place. You could have High Tea at the Lillie Langtry Bar, stay in the Oscar Wilde Suite, and the proprietress told guests the stories of those late Victorian days when the hotel was filled with the laughter of those pretty, young, high-living people.

We wondered: Was that her perfume, faint down the hallway? Did Wilde sit at this very table as he composed bon mots to entertain the Jersey Lillie? Was the bed we slept in the one that . . . ?

Though our travel agent was sending us to many more exciting places on that trip, we always remember it as the time we stayed at Lillie Langtry's hotel.

You see, we had put our European journey in the hands of a good travel agent, and, knowing our bent for history, he gave us that bonus. We had never heard of any of the hotels he put us into — and every one was an economical little jewel.

The point is, when you're going abroad, ask your travel agent to recommend places where you'd like to stay. Tell him your price range and any other requirements. Then — if you don't trust him implicitly — check out his choices in a good guide like Michelin's (see Chapter 4, Armchair Travel).

Use guidebooks like AAA's or Mobil's, also, to select an inn in the United States or Canada. The books describe locations, prices and facilities of almost every respectable hotel and motel in an area, as well as reservation phone numbers. The guidebooks also rate the inns for quality.

Check the guidebooks for facilities. It may be important to you to have a restaurant on the premises, or a swimming pool. Does it take pets? Is it air-conditioned? Does it have private baths? (Some older hotels don't.) Don't pay for fancy facilities you don't need — if you don't drink, why pay a premium to have a wetbar in your room, as classy as that might sound?

In addition to quality, cleanliness and price, here are some other things you'll want to know about your hotel or motel:

• Location — Is it where you want to be? The larger the city, the more important that is. If your next-day destination is Los Angeles International Airport, you don't want a hotel in mid-Wilshire, at least an hour's drive away. If you're going to London to see some plays, try to find a hotel reasonably near the West End theater district, or you might miss showtime. If you're not familiar with a city, get a map and plot the location of hotels you're considering against the attractions you want to see. AAA and American Express guides contain good city maps for that purpose. Of course, the closer you get to downtown or to major tourist attractions, the more you're likely to pay.

• Parking — If you're driving, is parking included in the room rate? Or do you have to pay extra? At downtown San Francisco hotels, typically, there's an extra $9-$20-a-night parking fee not stated in the guidebooks; rather, they'll note "overnight parking is available." Ask when you make reservations.

• Extra charges — Also find out, when you make reservations, whether the room rate includes taxes and service charges. Usually it doesn't, and local hotel taxes in some cities run as high as 20 percent.

WHAT THE RATINGS MEAN

In America, Mobil's five-star rating and AAA's five-diamond rating, printed in their guidebooks, are among the most coveted trophies in the innkeeping business, and few places rate that high. For the ordinary traveler, three-star and three-diamond places are just fine, thanks, and even one-star/diamond places are acceptable.

Both rating services have field agents who visit the inns and restaurants each year to update their ratings. We have found the commentaries and rating system of each of these guidebooks to be accurate and up-to-date. Similarly, *Michelin's Red Guide* ratings are the standard for overseas hotels.

But beware of directories and guidebooks put out by foreign governments or tourist agencies—some of their descriptions are on the optimistic side. And also look critically at descriptions of hotels in overseas-tour brochures — a "superior" hotel in one country might be described as "tourist-class" in another and a "dump" in the vernacular.

Reputable foreign tourism agencies use the hotel-classification system established by the Official Hotel and Resort Guide (OHRG), and your travel agent should be able to tell you whether a particular tour brochure is using those descriptions. Hotels are rated from "Superior Deluxe" (the best) to "Moderate Tourist Class" (stay away). Descriptions used in the OHRG system are at the end of this chapter.

SHOPPING FOR DISCOUNTS

You can make reservations at any major hotel or motel by dialing that chain's toll-free 800 number. But sometimes you'll save pennies and cost yourself dollars that way. Often the registration clerks on these nation-wide switchboards are not informed about deals offered by their local franchises.

Travel columnist Peter Greenberg (*The Savvy Traveler*) tells about booking a specially priced "Golden Summer" deal for $59 through Hilton Hotels' nationwide switchboard, only to arrive and find the local Hilton had a $39-a-night special going. He found out by asking after he got to the front desk, "Got any rooms tonight?"

"Yessir, we do," said the clerk.

"What's your cheapest room?" asked Greenberg.

When the clerk told him the price, he said, "I'll take it — and you can tear up my previous reservation for $65."

Use the toll-free numbers to shop for rates, to get directories, to ask about facilities, to get the local franchise's phone number — even to make reservations. But Greenberg's point is:

Never stop shopping for a rate, even after you've got a reservation, even after you get there. And that goes especially for 49ers-plus. Don't stop until you have called at least three hotels everywhere you plan to visit. And do not make reservations at any inn that doesn't offer you at least a 10 per cent seniors' discount. To be sure you're getting a real discount, ask what the regular rate is, and compare.

Even if you are on a freewheeling trip — going where the muse takes you — and unable to make reservations in advance, there is still no reason to stay anywhere you cannot get a discount.

Always ask for the seniors' discount, whether or not it's posted or listed in a directory. Young, inexperienced counter people may forget to tell you about them.

When you call for a reservation, let the clerk know if the cost of the room is more important to you than a mountain view. That's also the time to ask about taxes, parking and the other questions mentioned above.

Find out when you can check in, and find out about the inn's policy on late checkouts — will you be charged a half-day rate, or even for a full day?

Ask about special rates, and make sure the clerk quotes you the room price. When you get to the inn, by the way, don't hesitate to ask about a lower rate than the one you've been quoted — central reservation clerks for major chains often aren't aware of special local rate promotions or seniors' discounts.

If you make a "guaranteed reservation" backed by a major credit card, the inn has to put you up. When you make reservations, ask for a written confirmation as evidence that you have that guarantee.

Many hotels get overbooked — sometimes guests extend their stays, sometimes the hotel deliberately sells too much space, hoping for cancellations. Even a written confirmation or an advance deposit won't guarantee you'll have a room waiting.

But if you have given the hotel your credit-card number and asked for a guaranteed reservation, they will hold the room for the entire night. If you phone to cancel by 6 p.m. local time (4 p.m. at resorts), you aren't charged — just make sure to get a cancellation number in case the hotel accidentally bills your account.

In the rare event your guaranteed room has been sold to someone else and there's no other room available, it's customary that the hotel finds you a free room at a comparable hotel, take you to that hotel and give you a free long-distance telephone call. Insist on it — remember, no matter how crowded the town is, there is always an unoccupied room somewhere being saved for the king of England or the president of the hotel chain.

To learn more about how innkeepers operate, get the booklet *Tips for Travelers*; send $1 and an addressed, business-size envelope with 45 cents postage to Communications Department, American Hotel & Motel Association, 1201 New York Ave., N.W., Washington DC ,20005.

SENIOR DISCOUNTS

In hotels and motels in the United States, Mexico and Canada, some of the published senior discounts range up to 50 percent (Howard Johnson, some Marriotts, Stouffers), and discounts of 15-to-25 percent are common. Some chains also offer 49ers-plus discounts at their restaurants (Days Inn, Marriott, Red Lion). And some will let grandkids stay free in your room. Some have rooms for non-smokers at no extra charge, and some for the hearing-impaired. But you must ask for these when you make reservations.

A few chains require you to join their clubs (Days Inn, Vagabond Inn, Hampton Inn). But you can usually fill out an application blank when you walk into the lobby and get the discount that night. Most inns simply accept your AARP or Mature Outlook card as proof you're a 49er-plus. You are likely to save more than the $5 cost of membership in AARP the first night you're on the road.

Typical of the club deals is Hilton Hotels', which has just started a "Senior HHonors" plan for anyone 60 or older and for retired people over 55. For $45 a year you join a club that entitles you to discounts worth up to 50 percent at participating Hiltons and 20 percent at most of their restaurants, and a host of bonuses and credits for frequent stays.

Independent operators are just as eager to extend special deals to seniors. A spot check of independents around the United States batted 1.000 in finding senior discounts. For example:

Knight's Inn, Wichita, Kan., ☎ 316/942-1341 gives 49ers-plus $2 off the regular room rate of $29. The Capitol Inn in Montgomery, Ala., ☎ 205/265-0541 also gives seniors $2 off. The historic Peery Hotel in Salt Lake City ☎ 801/521-4300 gives

49ers-plus 10 percent off — all you have to do is show a membership card in a national seniors' organization.

OTHER SPECIAL RATES

Aside from published senior-citizen discounts, you can get astonishing rate reductions on lodgings if you'll simply be there when the hotels and motels want you to be there.

Off-season is one of those times. Another is on certain days when the inns are typically empty. And another time, particularly at country motels, is late in the day when the "Vacancy" sign is still lit.

• **Off-season** — You'll never never get a break in the winter at any of the fancy resorts in the Southwest — not even a seniors' discount. But in the summer, in places like Palm Springs, and Scottsdale, high-priced resorts typically rent their $250 rooms for as little as $40-to-$60 a night. The Westways Resort in Phoenix, for example, charges $47 in the summer for a room it gets $78 for in the winter.

Sure, mid-day temperatures are scorching — often into the 100s — but early mornings and evenings are refreshingly cool, and the dry climate makes even the hottest hours more bearable. You can tee off for nine holes just before dawn — snooze, swim or read when it's hottest — and get back into the outdoors (nine more holes, maybe?) just before sundown.

It happens in Mexico, Florida and the Caribbean, too — though the summer heat is stickier there. One of the best deals for seniors we ever heard of was the summer rate at the Naples Beach Hotel & Golf Club in Florida: a room regularly priced at $90 a person or more (double occupancy) going in the summer for as little as $42 — and that included a free round of golf each day on the club's championship course. (Naples Beach Hotel & Golf Club, 851 Golf Shore Blvd. N., Naples, FL 33940; ☎ 800/237-7600, in Florida ☎ 800/282-7601).

Find out from your travel agent which resorts have the best deals.

• **Special days** — Hotels catering to business travelers usually are empty on weekends, and mature travelers can get all kinds of good deals then. On the other hand, if you're traveling midweek, look for deals at resort-area motels and hotels, which typically are full on weekends.

That Westways Resort, which cuts its rate in half during the summer, cuts it another 40 percent on weekdays — getting you that $78 room for only $28 for two people (Westways Resort, P.O. Box 41624, Valley of the Sun, Phoenix, AZ 85080; ☎ 602/582-3868).

New Compri Hotels, which cater to business travelers, give deep discounts on weekends — plus senior citizen rates. When the Compri opened near Chicago's O'Hare Airport, it charged $85-99 per person on weekdays, but only $59 per couple on weekends. The 15 percent seniors' discount brought that down to $50.15 — little more than one-quarter of the weekday rate. (☎ 800/426-6774 for a directory and reservations).

• **Late in the day** — If you haul in to a motel late in the day, and the "Vacancy" sign is still on, that means you're in a good bargaining position. The revenue from a room is lost forever if the room isn't filled, and the motel wants you there very badly. That's a good time to start acting like a camel trader. All you have to do is give the motel operator a reason to give you a discount:

"How much is the room?"

"I'm an AAA member. Can't you do any better than that?"

"Well, what about your commercial rate — isn't that a better rate?" (Use the term "commercial rate" as if you know what you're talking about. Motel chains make deals with private companies for reduced rates so that business travelers will stay there. Most individual motels have long ago lost track of which companies they have deals with, so if you can simply flash a business card from any company it will frequently get you the commercial discount.)

"That's still awfully high. Don't you have a room toward the back?"

And so on. Once you get the price down as low as you can, then zing them with: "My senior-citizen discount applies to that, doesn't it?"

HOTEL PHONES: EXPENSIVE SURPRISE

You're probably already used to hotels adding a 50-cent surcharge whenever you make a local phone call. Now more U.S.

hotels have adopted the European custom of adding whopping surcharges to the billing for long-distance calls — even when you direct-dial. In Europe, those surcharges are sometimes double and triple the regular long-distance charge.

One good way to avoid these charges is to go downstairs and use the pay phone.

AT&T used to reimburse hotels and motels 10-to-15 percent of long-distance billings to help inkeepers defray the cost of handling calls. That ended with deregulation, when some inns began recovering those rebates — and more — from guests.

Some hotel chains have company-wide policies limiting surcharges. Marriott, for example, limits the charge to $1.25 or less for direct-dialed interstate calls. But most chains leave it up to individual properties, and we have heard of add-ons of up to 30 percent in North America. In Europe, on the other hand, an American staying at a Hamburg hotel told United Press International he was charged $110 for a $20 seven-minute call to Rochester, N.Y. Because some hotels' equipment can't detect whether a call actually goes through, some travelers also report being billed surcharges for long-distance calls that yielded only busy signals or weren't answered.

When you check into a hotel or motel, either here or abroad, with plans to make some long-distance calls, avoid nasty surprises at check-out time by asking in advance whether the hotel levies a surcharge, and how much it is. Ask also whether it levies the surcharge on all calls or just operator-assisted calls.

If you don't want to pay it, use a telephone elsewhere to make your call — in the lobby, at the airport or on the street — or have relatives call you in your room at a pre-arranged time. Another alternative when you're traveling abroad is using one of two new international services:

• AT&T's USA Direct service lets you access a long-distance operator in America through a local number in 12 countries: Australia, Belgium, British Virgin Islands, Denmark, Finland, France, Hong Kong, the Netherlands, Sweden, Great Britain and some parts of Japan and West Germany. And the system is expanding rapidly.

Because the hotel switchboard records the USA Direct call as local, you avoid the hotel's long-distance surcharge. You give the U.S. operator the number you want to call and your AT&T

calling-card number. You pay at the operator-assisted international rate — $5 to $6 for a three-minute call from London, for example, or $9 to $10 from Sydney.

☎ Call 800/874-4000, ext. 344, and AT&T will send you a brochure and a wallet card with the local numbers from every location where the service is available. You must also have an AT&T calling-card — arrange that through your local telephone company.

• Quick Call USA is a new service from International Telecharge which also uses local numbers. You'll be connected with an English-speaking operator, who will take your major credit-card number and the U.S. number you want to call. Quick Call USA operates in Austria, the Caribbean, Denmark, France, Korea, the Netherlands, Sweden, Switzerland, Great Britain and West Germany.

You can only talk for three minutes, and rates are somewhat higher than those of USA Direct — but you'll still save the enormous hotel surcharges in places where USA Direct doesn't operate.

You don't have to join anything or take out an extra credit card to use Quick Call USA. Just write 108 S. Akard, Dallas, TX 75202 for a wallet card containing the overseas phone numbers before your trip.

SPECIAL VACATION LODGINGS

There's no law, of course, that you have to stay at a hotel or motel. There are all kinds of other places to lay your head, including some just for mature travelers:

• **Bed & Breakfast Inns** — B&Bs are everywhere you look in America and Europe. These are usually big, quaint houses where the owners actually live and care for guests. Even for a single night, you become part of the owner's family, and you're treated accordingly. You'll find B&Bs in tiny little towns, in cities, in the country — there are even dude ranch B&Bs. It's tempting to describe B&Bs as "low-cost" — they used to be. Now some of their rates seem comparable to nearby motels', especially in popular tourist areas.

An unusual B&B program just for 49ers-plus is the Evergreen B&B Club. You agree to put up other members in your home for

$10 to $15 a night, and you can stay in other members' homes at the same price when you're traveling. Annual dues are $50 a couple, $40 a single. There are more than 700 members, including six in Europe and others in New Zealand, Israel and Mexico. Write Evergreen Bed & Breakfast Club, 16 Village Green, No. 203, Crofton, MD 21114 ☎ phone 301/261-0180.

Usually, you have to find a B&B on your own—a travel agent won't help you, since B&Bs rarely pay commissions. There are hundreds of B&B associations, and hundreds of directories. Sometimes you can get one from the local tourism authority or chamber of commerce. Many B&B directories are available in bookstores. One good one is *Bed & Breakfast U.S.A.* by Betty Rundback and Nancy Kramer ($10.95, Dutton), giving rates, accommodations and prices for 981 B&Bs throughout the U.S. and Canada. The American B&B Association puts out a series of regional guidebooks ranging in price from $6 to $17.95; for a catalog, write the association at 16 Village Green, No.203, Crofton, MD 21114. A computerized reservation system for 35,000 guesthouses in Europe is European Tourist Information, 1300 Dove St., Newport Beach, CA 92660 (☎ 800/621-1934, in California 714/851-1787).

The 320-page *InnServ Reservation Guidebook IV* describes more than 650 U.S. B&Bs. Buy the directory for $9.95 and get a free quarterly B&B newsletter, *InnTouch*. Write InnServ, Rt. 1, Box 47, Redkey, IN 47373 (☎ 800/222-3209, in Indiana 317/369-2245).

• **Paradors, pousadas, castles and manors** — Spain has turned some of its finest old castles and monasteries into housing for travelers, called "paradors." Rates for a couple are as low as $50 a night, including breakfast. For information and a list of paradors, write the Spanish National Tourist Office, 665 Fifth Ave., New York, NY 10022 ☎ 212/759-8822. In neighboring Portugal, the same kind of accommodations are called "pousadas," and rates are even lower than at paradors. Write the Portuguese National Tourist Office, 548 Fifth Ave., New York, NY 10036 ☎ 212/354-4403.

French chateaux, on the other hand, are strictly luxury class — you can stay in one for $100 to $140 a night. Write the French Government Tourist Office, 610 Fifth Ave., New York, NY 10020 ☎ 212/757-1125.

There are 55 castle-hotels, called "schlosse", throughout the scenic countryside of West Germany. They cost as little as $45 a night. Get the booklet *Gast Im Schloss* free from the German National Tourist Office, 747 Third Ave., New York, NY 10017 ☎ 212/308-3300. Thirty castle-hotels open their doors to tourists in Austria. Write Austrian National Tourist Office, 500 Fifth Ave., New York, NY 10110 ☎ 212/697-0651.

British castles are pretty expensive, but there are a few open overnight to tourists. At British country manor houses, on the other hand, overnights are ranging around $60. Get the booklet *BTA Commended Country Hotels, Guest Houses and Restaurants* from any British Tourist Authority office.

A Relais & Chateaux Association has as members 372 former castles, abbeys and manor houses that accept guests — half in France, the rest in 36 other countries. Get the *Relais & Chateaux Guide* from Mitchell Tours, 200 Madison Ave., New York, NY 10016 ☎ 800/372-1323, in N.Y. 212/696-1323. Mitchell also packages relais and chateaux tours.

• **Hosted holidays** — You can stay in the home of a foreign couple at little cost. Only if you want to, you can host them in return.

The Senior Travel Exchange Program (STEP) claims to hold the cost of European trips 40% percent below comparable commercial programs. The key is "hosting," housing visitors with host families for part of the trip.

A recent 18-day tour of Austria cost under $1,995, including air from New York, San Francisco and Los Angeles gateways. It featured hosting by two different families for six days each and six days in Vienna, including meals and sightseeing. Hosting families offered bed and breakfast, plus some other meals and sightseeing throughout northern Austria. STEP books 35 to 40 people on each tour, both singles and couples.

There were similar tours in Germany and Great Britain. Six month's advance booking is required so hosts can be found for the tour dates. And, since STEP is run by volunteers, there's a $3 handling charge to get a brochure with trip details. Write Senior Travel Exchange Program, P.O. Box H, Santa Maria, CA 93456, or ☎ call 805/925-5743.

The Evergreen Bed & Breakfast Club, discussed earlier, is another hosting program open only to mature travelers.

• **House swaps** — You simply trade houses with a family living where you want to visit. Start at least six months in advance of your trip, and keep your dates loose, for it usually takes that long to get arrangements synchronized for two families who don't really know each other — both families have to travel at the same time, of course. Agencies dealing with house swaps publish directories, which they sell you; then you arrange the swap directly. They include Vacation Exchange Club, 12006 111th Ave., Youngtown, AZ 85363, ☎ 602/972-2186, 6,000 listings in 40 countries, $15 per issue; Interservice Home Exchange, P.O. Box 87, Glen Echo, MD 20812, ☎ 301/229-7567, 1,000 listings including yours, $24; and International Home Exchange Service, P.O. Box 3975, San Francisco, CA 94119, ☎ 415/435-3497, 500 listings, including yours, $45.

Among agencies that will arrange house swaps for you are Home Exchange International, 22713 Ventura Blvd., Suite F, Woodland Hills, CA 91364, ☎ 213/992-8990; At Home Abroad, Sutton Town House, 405 E. 56th St., Suite 6-H, New York, NY 10022, ☎ 212/421-9165; and Caribbean Home Rentals, Box 710, Palm Beach, FL 33480, ☎ 305/833-4454.

• **Self-catered homes** — On a "self-catered holiday," you simply rent somebody's vacant house. These comfortable family lodgings are now offered throughout the European countryside, as well as in some cities, including London and Paris.

A recent traveler reports costs of $36 a night, including gas and lights, for a Paris studio near the Louvre; $33 a night for three rooms just off Baker Street in London, including utilities, a weekly linen change and a color TV.

Among agencies handling self-catered holidays are Alamo, P.O. Box 936, Alamo, CA 94507, ☎ 415/935-7065; Eastone Overseas Accommodations, 225 Andover Rd., Sparta, NJ 07871; Elysees-Concorde, 9 rue Royale, Paris, France 75008; and Holiday Flats Ltd., 51 Kensington Ct., Kensington, London W8, England.

• **Vacation apartments** — These are for longer stays. You have a chance to settle into the neighborhood, make friends with the fishmonger and get an insider's look at the country. Costs are lower, too — as low as $25 a night for some programs, including sightseeing and airfare. AARP, Saga Tours and Grand Circle Tours all have apartment programs abroad.

Another vacation-apartment plan is run by Oakwood Resort Apartments, with 60 locations in the West as well as Washington, North Carolina, Virginia and Atlanta. In winters, travelers over 54 who stay 30 days get one-third off regular rates, which range from $797/month in Houston to $1,510 in Los Angeles. For a directory and reservations, call ☎ 800/421-6654.

• **College housing** — More than 500 colleges and universities around the world make their empty dorms available to travelers for $6 to $16 a night. They're listed in the *U.S. and Worldwide Accommodations Guide*. Send $9.95 to Campus Travel Service, P.O. Box 5007, Laguna Beach, CA 92652.

IN SUMMARY:

— Never pay full rates for lodgings, no matter where you travel in the United States, Canada and Mexico. Always ask for the senior discount.

— Travel off-season and on weekends for better rates.

— Check guidebooks to find the location of your hotel, and plot it on city maps.

— Beware of the hotel's long-distance-telephone surcharges.

— Consider unusual kinds of lodging that can save you money.

★ ★ ★
Travel Tool
★ ★ ★

HOTELS AND MOTELS OFFERING DISCOUNTS FOR 49ERS-PLUS

Rates and deals listed here are subject to change, but use this survey as a guide to shopping for the best senior citizen discounts available.

Clarion
— See Quality Inns.

Comfort Inns
— See Quality Inns.

Compri Hotels
— New hotel group in several major U.S. cities, catering to businessmen, give 15 per cent off on all rates, plus full breakfasts to AARP members and other seniors over 60 .
☎ 800/426-6774.

Days Inns
— September Days Club has discounts of 10-50 percent for 49ers-plus and discounts on car rentals and local attractions. Most of the 400 inns in 42 states also give AARP members 10-15 percent off, and grandkids eat free at many Days Inns restaurants.
☎ 800/325-2525.

Econo Lodges and Econo-Travel Motor Hotels
— About 95 percent of the 400 lodges in 40 states give AARP members 10 percent off.
☎ 800-446-6900.

Hampton Inns
— Lifestyle 50 program for 49ers-plus permits up to four people in a room for the price of one at each of 150 inns across the country. Free membership. Also offers non-smoking rooms and rooms for the hearing-impaired.
☎ 800/426-7866 (TDD number is ☎ 800/451-4833).

Harley Hotels
— Offer 10 percent senior discounts at 20 properties, but not at the Harley flagship hotel in New York.
☎ 800/321-2323.

Hilton Hotels
— Senior HHonors Club, for those 60 and older and retired people over 54, costs $45/year ($75/lifetime), entitles members to lodging discounts up to 50 percent at more than 200 participating Hiltons and 20 percent off at most Hilton restaurants, additional frequent-traveler discounts, member discounts on Hertz car rentals and other perks.
Write Hilton Senior HHonors Service Center, 2050 Chennault Dr., Carrollton, TX 75006, ☎ or phone 214/239-0511.

Hospitality Inns
— Includes 200 Master Hosts Inns and Resorts and Red Carpet Inns. 10 percent off regular rates only at participating locations.
☎ 800/251-1962.

Holiday Inns
— Senior Savings program offers 10 percent off to 49ers-plus only at participating inns.
☎ 800/465-4329.

Howard Johnson
— Road Rally Club gives 15 percent discounts to those over 59 and members of any national seniors' organization. Some HoJos offer up to 50 percent off with advance reservations Club also gives discount coupons and holds monthly sweepstakes drawings.
☎ 800/634-3464.

La Quinta Motor Inns
— 200 inns in 29 states give 15 percent off, except for some blackout dates, to travelers over 55 and members of national seniors organizations.
☎ 800/531-5900.

L-K Penny Pincher Inns
— 10 percent off to AARP members, or anyone over 54.
☎ 800/848-5767 (in Ohio 800/282-5711).

Marriott
— Leisurelife Program for those over 62 gives 50 percent discounts at three-fourths of the 130 worldwide locations, as well as 25 percent off at their restaurants. Even non-participating Marriotts may give AARP members 50 percent discounts.
☎ 800/228-9290.

Master Hosts Inns and Resorts
— See Hospitality Inns.

Nendels Motor Inns
— See Vagabond Motor Inns

Omni International
— 37 Omnis around the country give 50 percent discounts to AARP members, plus 15 percent off meals.
☎ 800/228-2121.

Quality International
— 600 Quality Inns, Royale Hotels, Comfort and Clarion properties give 30 percent discounts to members of AARP and of United's Silver Wings Plus program (for travelers over 60). Other seniors over 55 get 10 percent discounts. You have to book 30 days in advance, and deposits are non-refundable. Non-smoking rooms available.
☎ Reserve through 800/228-LUNG and $2 goes to American Lung Associationn. Regular reservation number is 800/228-5050 (TDD phone 800/228-3323).

Radisson Hotels
— More than 100 Radissons around the country give 49ers-plus 25 percent off.
☎800/228-9822.

Red Carpet Inns
— See Hospitality Inns.

Red Roof Inns
— 10 percent discounts to guests 60 and over.
☎ 800/843-7663.

Red Lion Inns
— Prime Rate Discount program at most of the 59 Red Lions and Thunderbird Inns in the West give 49ers-plus 20 percent on rooms and 15 percent off at restaurants.
☎ 800/547-8010.

Rodeway Inns
— 150 inns in the U.S. and Canada give AARP members and anyone else over 55 10 percent off all year. Some offer bigger discounts.
☎ 800/228-2000 (402/496-0101 from Nebraska, Alaska and Mexico).

Royale Hotels
— See Quality International.

Sandman Motels
— See Vagabond Inns.

Scottish Inns
— See Hospitality Inns.

Sheraton
— Sheraton Retired Persons Plan gives 25 percent discounts for travelers over 60 and AARP members on some rooms on most dates at 480 worldwide locations. Grandkids stay free in your room. Sheratons along I-95 offer AARP members even deeper discounts. ☎ 800/325-3535.

Stouffer
— Some properties — not the resorts — take part in the $59-or-less Great Years rate for those over 60. Discounts can range up to 50 percent.
☎800/465-4329 to ask about individual locations.

Thunderbird Inns
— See Red Lion Inns.

Travelodge
— 450 Travelodge and Viscount Hotels give 15 percent off to AARP members all year. The chain's Super Saver rates (for everyone) apply, if lower. Grandkids under 18 stay free in the same room.
☎ 800/255-3050.

Vagabond Inns
— 100-plus Vagabond Inns (Southwest), Nendels Motor Inns (Northwest) and Sandman Motels (Canada) offer Club 55 discounts averaging 15 percent, plus discounts on trips and social events. Membership for travelers over 55 is $10. Grandkids stay free in your room.
☎ 800/543-3455 for Vagabonds, 800/547-0106 for Nendels,
800/663-6900 for Sandman.

Viscount Hotels
— See Travelodge.

★ ★ ★
Travel Tool
★ ★ ★

OVERSEAS HOTEL CLASSIFICATIONS

Here are terms used in the hotel-classification system of the Official Hotel and Resort Guide (OHRG), which is the standard used in reputable overseas guidebooks and tour brochures. Not all countries, however, accept these standard definitions:

Superior Deluxe — Among the world's top hotels. An exclusive and expensive luxury hotel, often palatial, offering the highest standards of service, accommodations and facilities.

Deluxe — An outstanding property offering many of the same features as Superior Deluxe, except in some cases a small number of minimum-rated accommodations may be of inferior grade. May be less grand and offer more reasonable rates. "Safe to recommend to the most discriminating clients,"says OHRG.

Moderate Deluxe — Basically a Deluxe hotel, but with qualifications. Hotel may be a well-established famous name, depending heavily on past reputation, some accommodations or public areas may not be up to Deluxe standards. If modern, the hotel may be heavily marketed to business clients, with fine accommodations and public rooms offering Deluxe standards in comfort, but lacking in atmosphere or personal service. "May be overpriced."

Superior First Class — An above-average hotel. May be an exceptionally well-maintained older hotel, more often a superior modern hotel specifically designed for first-class market. Accommodations and public areas are expected to be tastefully furnished and very comfortable. "In most cases will satisfy the discriminating clients."

First Class — An average, comfortable hotel. The majority of accommodations are good, although some may be below First Class standards. May have some Deluxe rooms or suites. Public areas are standard, usually nothing special. "Should be satisfactory for better groups."

Moderate First Class — Basically a First-Class establishment, slightly below average. Generally, has comfortable, simple accommodations and public areas, though not always kept up to standards. Some of the rooms . . . may tend to be small and functional. "Suitable for cost-conscious clients."

Superior Tourist Class — Primarily a budget property with mostly well-kept, functional accommodations, some up to First Class standards. Public rooms may be limited or non-existent. Often just a place to sleep, but may have some charming or intimate features. "May be a good value. Will satisfy clients on a budget . . . or student groups."

Tourist Class — Strictly a budget operation, with some facilities or features of Superior Tourist Class. "Should generally be used with caution," warns OHRG.

Moderate Tourist Class — Low-budget operations, often quite old and may not be well-kept. "Should only be used in a pinch if no others are available."

★ ★ ★
Travel Tool
★ ★ ★

LODGING TERMS YOU SHOULD KNOW

American Plan (AP) — Also called "full-board," "full-pension" and "full American" plans. A room whose price includes three meals a day — whether you eat them or not. They are usually fixed-price meals with limited choice of entrees.

Continental Plan — A room whose rates include a light breakfast and no other meals. The continental breakfast usually is only coffee plus rolls or bread, no juice.

Double Occupancy — A room that is shared by two people, whether it is priced per person or per night. It can have twin beds or any size of single bed.

European Plan (EP) — Room only.

Housekeeping Plan — A room or suite that has a kitchenette stocked with cooking and eating utensils, but not food.

Modified American Plan (MAP) — Also called "half-board," "half-pension" or "demi-pension." A room whose price includes two meals a day, usually breakfast and diner.

Ocean Front — A room directly facing the ocean.

Ocean View — A room from which it's possible to see the ocean, usually on the side of the hotel.

Pension — In Europe, a guesthouse or a small inn.

Single Room — A room with one bed for one person.

Single Room Supplement — Difference in price between half of a twin room and the actual price of a single room.

Twin Room — A room with two beds for two people.

Voucher — A proof of pre-payment, usually issued by a travel agent or hotel chain.

NOTES

CHAPTER 6

MONEY MATTERS

Here's How to Sort Through Foreign Currency

I f you want to travel abroad, you talk to a travel agent. If you want to play the international money markets, you buy a seat on the Chicago Mercantile Exchange.

But don't get the two confused. Whether the English pound is $1.66 or $1.68 today should not alter your decision on how to buy pounds for your trip to London, or how to carry them. You are traveling for pleasure, not playing the international money market.

If you're traveling abroad, however, you do need to understand something about foreign exchange — otherwise you could end up paying too much for things, or pass up real bargains because the price seems too high.

UNDERSTANDING FOREIGN EXCHANGE

The "foreign exchange rate" simply is the amount of foreign money you get in exchange for a U.S. dollar. The rates are established by currency traders on international money markets and by actions of international banks. The rates published in your local newspaper or *The Wall Street Journal* are the "international bank rates," the rates at which banks trade billions of dollars with each other. If you're trading only $100 worth of U.S. dollars for $100 worth of British pounds, expect the exchange rate to be 1-to-4 percent less favorable than the one you saw published.

And the rate published tomorrow may be several pence different, yet — better or worse — than today's.

Don't worry about it. Over the course of a month, the rate for U.S. dollars against any major international currency rarely fluctuates more than $10 on $1,000.

What you do need to know is that a British pound costs roughly $1.70(US), for example, or that you get a little more than 6 French francs for $1. And often, when you're bargaining at a flea market or trying to figure out whether you're getting gouged at a restaurant, you need to be able to do that math quickly.

Electronic conversion calculators are a good way to do that. Those we've seen fit in your pocket and range in price from $5 to $21. You program the current exchange rate for whatever country you're visiting, and the calculator converts the price you're looking at into dollars. You can buy a conversion calculator almost anywhere electronic calculators are sold and at many foreign currency dealers.

There are also mechanical calculators, cheaper but not as easy to use — in effect, currency slide rules.

At the end of this chapter is a different kind of conversion table, one based on approximate conversion rates designed to help you with the math.

THE 'PARALLEL MARKETS'

In some countries where local currency is weak or fluctuates wildly, in addition to the official exchange rate there is a "parallel market" — the rate you can get on the street by paying in U.S. dollars instead of the local currency. In countries where the exchange rate is officially controlled, it's called the "black market" and using it can get you jailed.

Some friends who recently visited Moscow admired a street painter's charcoal sketch of a cathedral. It was priced in rubles at the equivalent of $140. How much if we pay in dollars? they asked. The reply was, "$20." It's dangerous to bargain that way in any Soviet bloc country. The Soviet Union restricts the amount of dollars its citizens can take out, but encourages anything that brings dollars in, so our friends might not have been jailed, if caught. But they'd have slept better in Moscow if they'd just paid the rubles.

Some countries control their currencies by restricting the amount you can enter or leave with. India, for instance, prohibits the import or export of rupees.

In Israel and the rest of the Middle East, U.S. dollars — and even personal checks — will buy much more on the legal parallel market than either traveler's checks or credit cards. Check with a foreign currency dealer, at the consulates of countries you're planning to visit or with your travel agent to find out whether there's a legal parallel market and whether there are restrictions on the amount of dollars you can bring in and local currency you can bring out.

And before you buy currency to take into a foreign country, ask whether that's legal. You can buy rupees at foreign exchange offices in New York City, for example — but if you don't ask about India's restrictions, some dealers may not volunteer the information.

CARRYING CASH ABROAD

Where the laws permit — and that's most places overseas — you should arrive with at least a few units of the local currency in your pocket and a low-cost way to get more of them.

Once we learned that the hard way. We had bused over from Munich that afternoon, and were scheduled to spend only two hours in Strasbourg, France, before getting on the Rhine boat for a cruise back through Germany. No need to purchase any francs for such a short stay, we thought — besides, most border cities accept the currency of both countries, and we had lots of marks.

France is famous for its public toilets — their frequency, their cleanliness and their nosy attendants. And when we needed to use one badly in Strasbourg, it was nearby, below the town square. But it was a coin-op — you needed centimes to open the door. And, for once, there was no attendant in sight. We discovered, to our dismay, that German pfennigs don't fit in French coin slots.

For 15 minutes we waited, standing first on one foot and then the other. When the attendant finally returned, she spoke only French. We held out a handful of German coins, gestured wildly at the toilet doors, and took an extra precious five minutes getting her to understand what we wanted.

Finally, she selected some coins from our palm, walked over and unlocked one of the doors with a key, standing aside while we rushed in.

Never again would we arrive in France without francs.

THE STARTER PACK

You need cash the instant you arrive — to tip the porter, to rent a baggage cart, to catch a cab or a bus to your hotel, to make a phone call, to tip the bellboy, to open the pay-toilet. Neither credit cards nor travelers checks will work. And, except for friendly places like Mexico and Canada, the U.S. dollar is not nearly as appreciated nor as acceptable as the local currency.

Don't count on the airport's foreign exchange window being open when you arrive, either — it could be too early, a weekend or a holiday. Bring along enough foreign currency to get you started, to last until downtown banks are open or at least until you can get to your hotel.

U.S. banks no longer package "Tip Packs" — those neat little $10 packets of foreign coins and currency in various denominations you could buy for something like $10.50. Currency values fluctuate too wildly these days to package up cash and leave it sitting on a shelf, bankers tell us.

But you need to make up your own "Tip Packs" before you go. Some banks in large cities still handle small foreign-exchange amounts for customers who need pocket money abroad. Or visit a foreign exchange firm like Deak International, with 60 offices throughout the country, or other currency-exchange specialists listed in the Yellow Pages. Some travel agencies, like American Express Travel Services, sell foreign currency. International airports in the United States also have foreign-exchange windows.

If you don't live near any of these, you can order foreign currency by mail from Deak International. Get a cashier's check in dollars from your bank made out to "Deak International," mail it to Deak at 160 Franklin St., Boston, MA 02110, along with a cover letter specifying the nation's currency you want. Deak will do the conversion and send you the currency by registered mail. The cost is $9 for up to $1,000 worth of foreign currency. Be sure to allow plenty of lead time for your payment to clear and for the money to arrive at your home.

If you're going on a cruise to a foreign port, getting the local currency is easier — the ship's purser office will handle foreign exchange, where it's required.

How much foreign cash should you carry? Though the answer varies from country to country, you'll be told you'll get a better exchange rate — more foreign currency for your U.S. dollar — over there than you will over here. Therefore, most authorities say, you should arrive with just enough foreign cash to meet your minimum needs and plan to get more at a downtown bank.

We disagree. We think the problems you'll encounter if you arrive without enough cash are not worth the few pence or centimes you save by waiting to purchase your currency abroad.

If you customarily walk around at home with $50 to $100 in your pocket, it makes sense that you should do the same abroad — arriving with $50 to $100 in foreign currency in your pocket. Even more, in fact, because generally things cost more abroad. And, just as you would at home, carry at least $20 of it in small bills and change.

GETTING MORE CASH ABROAD

Taking cash abroad and getting some more when you need it are becoming easier. Now if you carry a standard U.S.-based credit card, you can operate thousands of automatic teller machines (ATMs) around the world to get a cash advance just as if they were at your branch bank around the corner. And these ATMs dispense the local currency.

They make it unnecessary to carry around large wads of bills, which if stolen cannot be replaced. They also make it unnecessary to carry large amounts of traveler's checks.

In addition to ATMs, you can use your Visa, MasterCard, American Express card or Diners Club card to draw cash or cash checks at banks almost anywhere in the world.

To use ATMs, you need a special card and a Personal Identification Number (PIN). Before you go, phone your credit-card company (there's a toll-free 800 number on every bill you receive) to apply for an ATM card and a list of overseas locations where you can get cash.

Use your credit card, also, whenever you can at stores, restaurants, hotels and the like that do not charge you a premium for using it. The exchange rate will be better than you can get anywhere else officially because it's figured by your credit-card company at the international bank rate.

Write down the number of your credit-card account and keep it in a safe place — not in your wallet where you carry the credit card. That way, if your credit card is lost or stolen overseas you can alert your credit-card company right away. That will limit your liability if someone uses your card to go on a shopping binge. But it will not necessarily get your card replaced before the end of your trip, as traveler's checks might be.

TRAVELER'S CHECKS

You still need to carry traveler's checks for places that simply don't take credit cards, or to use if your credit card is lost.

Do you remember when you could cash a traveler's check almost anywhere at face value? Well, in the United States, you still can. But many places overseas nowadays charge an "encashment fee" of up to 8 percent — exchange rates aside. That's too much. For that reason, while you still have to carry traveler's checks, you should cash them only as a last resort.

Typically, U.S. banks charge 1 percent when you buy traveler's checks, and cash in any leftovers free. Preferred customers at some banks even get traveler's checks without any commission, as do AAA members, and Deak International offices also sell U.S. and foreign traveler's checks without commission. Overseas, you can still cash them free at offices of the issuing company — you can cash American Express traveler's checks at six AmEx offices in London, for example, and get the best exchange rate, to boot, for turning them into pounds. But other places are likely to charge you that whopping encashment fee.

When you buy traveler's checks before your trip, it's a good idea to ask the seller for a list of overseas places where the checks can be cashed free.

If you have to cash a traveler's check, the best place to cash it usually is at a downtown bank rather than at the airport, your hotel or at a restaurant — the exchange rate, supposedly, is better.

Actually, we feel the convenience factor is worth 3 or 4 points — if the place where you want to cash your traveler's check doesn't charge more than 3 or 4 percent above the published international bank rate, go ahead and cash it. Don't spend half your vacation shopping for the best rate.

One way to avoid that exchange-rate worry is to buy your U.S. traveler's checks denominated in the foreign currency — that is, buy your checks in pounds or francs in the beginning. Deak, Thomas Cook, American Express and any number of foreign banks doing business in this country sell traveler's checks denominated in foreign currency units. You can cash these at face value almost anywhere in the country you're visiting. Even so, you may still have to pay some kind of encashment fee.

Traveler's checks are still one of the safest ways to carry large amounts of money overseas. If they are lost or stolen, no one can cash them but you. And if you have written down the serial numbers of your checks, they can be replaced by the issuing company usually within 24 hours, no matter where in the world you are.

Our advice to travelers is to use your credit card whenever you can. And carry an emergency supply — say, $1,000 or so — in traveler's checks which you do not plan to use. That's enough to tide you over should your credit cards get lost.

When you get home, if you cash in your traveler's checks at your hometown bank where you bought them, it will have cost you next to nothing to carry them.

OVERSEAS VOUCHERS

Another new way to pay for things when you travel overseas is with vouchers — in effect, prepayment for items like rental cars, hotel rooms and tours — before you leave home.

Overseas voucher programs are being promoted by Visa, MasterCard and Citicorp, among others, and sold through some travel agents. In making out your travel itinerary, your travel agent prepares a voucher good for so many nights at a given hotel, for example, and makes out a charge slip against your credit card. That guarantees the rates — the exchange rate as well as the room rate.

You present the voucher when you check in to your hotel — it's a confirmation slip for your reservation, as well as evidence you've already paid.

Vouchers are refundable at face value if you don't use the service. They're not transferable — they can't be used by anybody but you — and if they're lost or stolen, they're replaceable just like a traveler's check.

Other credit card companies are starting to explore the voucher idea, which they say could amount to a $16 billion industry, and soon most travel agents will be able to offer them for some overseas services.

So long as it doesn't cost you anything extra, we feel the voucher system is another good way to pay for your overseas travels because it means just that much less cash or traveler's checks to carry.

GETTING EMERGENCY CASH

If you run out of cash while traveling, the quickest way to get some is to use your credit card, as we said above.

But if you don't carry a credit card, there's always Western Union and the good old U.S. Consulate.

If you're out of cash abroad, call friends back home and ask them to go to a Western Union office and send you an International Money Order.

They can phone Western Union if they have a credit card to charge it against — ☎ toll-free 800/325-4176. Your friend must give Western Union details on where the money is to be sent — your name, city, bank and branch.

You'll get the money a little quicker at the nearest American consulate. Have Western Union make the money order payable to the Department of State and send it to the Citizens Emergency Center, Room 4811, 2201 C St. N.W., Washington, DC 20520, ☎ 202/632-5225. Include in the wire your name, the name of the consular office overseas where you'll pick up the money and sender's name and address.

The same method works, by the way, if you run out of cash while you're traveling in the United States.

OUR BORDER BUDDIES

If you're making only short trips into Mexico or Canada, don't worry about exchanging dollars (US) for dollars (CDN) or for pesos. Just know the exchange rates. For years, the rate up north has been $3(US) for $4(CDN), and lately has gone up to approximately $4(US) for $5(CDN).

Merchants in U.S. border cities, as well as most resorts, accept the Canadian dollar at the exchange rate or better, and Canadian merchants gladly take U.S. dollars at the going rate. The dollar, as much as the peso, is the local currency in Mexican border cities and resort areas. U.S. credit cards and traveler's checks are accepted in both Mexico and Canada.

The U.S. dollar is accepted as trading currency on most Caribbean islands, as well, though you can buy some Caribbean currencies before you leave the United States for considerably less than you can in the islands.

RETURNING WITH CHANGE

You don't have to spend all your local currency before you leave a country. Leave yourself enough for taxi fare, airport tips and perhaps a drink or a candy bar at the airport.

Some countries also require you to pay an airport tax in the local currency. Allow for that, too, or you could wind up sitting in the waiting room watching your plane leave without you.

After those last-minute needs are satisfied, simply trade in what's left over for the local currency of the next country you're going to visit — or bring it home and exchange it right at the airport foreign exchange window. You won't lose anything on the exchange except for the coins.

Coins are cumbersome to handle and convert, and many exchange facilities won't even touch them. At Dulles airport near Washington and at a few other international airports, relief agencies solicit foreign coins from passengers returning from abroad to finance their projects.

Another thing you can do with your foreign coins, far more valuable than turning them in, is to give them to your grand kids as mementos of your trip.

IN SUMMARY:

— Always know the local exchange rate and how to convert prices into dollars.

— Never arrive overseas without some local currency in your pocket.

— To use your traveler's checks overseas, you are likely to be charged an "encashment fee" ranging up to 8 per cent.

— As a money strategy, carry about $100 worth of local currency; use credit cards and vouchers whenever you can to pay for goods and services and get new cash; and carry only an emergency supply of traveler's checks — but try not to use them.

★ ★ ★
Travel Tool
★ ★ ★

CONVERTING FOREIGN CURRENCY

Here's how to handle the math for converting foreign currencies or prices into U.S. dollar amounts. The table is based on approximate foreign exchange rates in early 1989. Here's an example: With Argentine australs selling for approximately 2 1/2¢, you'd get 40 for $1. Therefore, divide Argentine prices by 40 to determine dollar equivalents. A 4,000 austral sweater, for instance, would cost you $100. Before you go, check your math against the prevailing exchange rates the week you leave, which you can find listed in *The Wall Street Journal* and many major dailies.

To convert into dollars from:

Argentine Australs	Divide by 40.
Australian Dollars	Divide by 1.2.
Austrian Schillings	Divide by 13.
Belgian Francs	Divide by 40.
Brazilian Cruzados	Even
British Pounds	Multiply by 1.7.
Canadian Dollars	Divide by 1.2.
Chinese Yunan	Divide by 4.
Danish Kroner	Divide by 7.

Dutch Guilders	Divide by 2.
Finnish Markkas	Divide by 4.5.
French Francs	Divide by 6.
Greek Drachmas	Divide by 160.
Hong Kong Dollars	Divide by 8.
Indian Rupees	Divide by 15.
Israeli Shekels	Divide by 1.8.
Italian Lire	Divide by 1,400.
Japanese Yen	Divide by 130.
Mexican Pesos	Divide by 2400
New Zealand Dollars	Divide by 1.6.
Norwegian Krone	Divide by 7.
Philippines Pesos	Divide by 20.
Portuguese Escudos	Divide by 155.
Russian Rubles	Divide by 5.
Singapore Dollars	Divide by 2.
South African Rands	Divide by 2.5.
South Korean Won	Divide by 700
(or multiply by 13 and subtract four zeros).	
Spanish Pesetas	Divide by 120.
Swedish Kroner	Divide by 6.
Taiwanese Dollar	Divide by 30.
Thai Bahts	Divide by 25.
Turkish Liras	Divide by 2,000
West German Marks	Divide by 2.

NOTES

CHAPTER 7

YOUR PAPERS, PLEASE

The Paperwork Blizzard Should Start Early

N o matter where you go overseas, you need a passport. And that's just the start of the paperwork blizzard that may take months to dig through.

You may need a visa, too.

You need a wallet full of other documents, as well: special papers to shop, papers to drive, papers for your medicine, even papers for your Japanese-made camera.

And don't forget papers that list your traveler's check numbers, your credit-card numbers, your emergency phone numbers and your itinerary.

And leave room for even more papers — you'll probably bring back more paperwork from overseas than you start out with.

Here's how to make it through the paperwork blizzard:

GETTING A PASSPORT

The passport is that 3 1/2-by-5-inch blue booklet with the impressive seal on the front that is proof to foreign governments you're a citizen in good standing. It also gets you back into the country when you return.

Canada and Mexico are the only countries we know of that you can conveniently visit for more than a few days without having a U.S. passport. Even the few countries that don't require you to have a passport do require some proof of citizenship — and a passport is the best evidence you can use.

Jamaica, for example, doesn't require you to have a passport or a visa — just a tourist card that you get free at the airport when you arrive. But to get the tourist card, you have to show proof of citizenship and a photo. And it's often less bother to carry a passport than to track down a long-lost birth certificate. A list of countries that don't require passports for travelers from the United States is at the end of this chapter.

Apply for your passport as far in advance as you can. In the spring, when applications are heaviest, it can take months to get a passport issued.

Start by getting two new 2-by-2-inch photos of yourself — color or black-and-white. Just visit any instant-print shop or commercial studio that advertises passport-photo service. If you need visas (see next section), get extra prints made, too. If you'll be gone more than a few day, carry some extra photos with you in case your passport is lost or stolen; it will expedite replacement.

If you've never had a U.S. passport, you need to appear personally at any of 13 U.S. Passport Agencies — in Boston, Chicago, Honolulu, Houston, Los Angeles, Miami, New Orleans, New York, Philadelphia, San Francisco, Seattle, Stamford, Conn., and Washington — or at one of the 3,500 post offices or county clerks' offices that take passport applications. When you go, bring these documents:

- A completed passport application form (DSP-11).
- Proof of citizenship: your naturalization papers or a birth certificate. If you don't have a birth certificate, write the Public Health Office, c/o Vital Statistics Department, of the state where you were born. If the record's been destroyed, get a letter from the Secretary of State or State Registrar that no record exists; then take that, along with a baptismal certificate, hospital birth record or insurance policy as proof that you were born in the United States.
- Personal identification. A driver's license will do, or something like an employment ID card that has your photo and signature.
- Those two photos.
- Payment. Your first passport will cost $42.

Every individual who's traveling with you needs a separate passport. If you plan to travel with grandchildren, they need passports, too. But the cost for them is only $27.

If you're renewing your passport, you can apply by mail. You need to renew if your passport was issued more than 12 years ago. Get a Form DSP-82 at any U.S. Passport Office, courthouse, post office or even your travel agent. Send it to the passport agency nearest you, along with two new 2-by-2-inch photos, your old passport and a check or money order for $35.

If your passport is lost in the United States, report it to the nearest passport agency. If it's stolen, also tell the local police. If it's lost overseas, report it to the local U.S. consulate or embassy and to the police. If you have ID and can prove you're a U.S. citizen, you'll get a new passport quickly. For handy proof, tuck away a photocopy of your passport's data page in a separate, safe place.

TOURIST VISAS

A visa stamped on your passport represents a foreign government's permission for you to enter and travel in its country. You get a visa by writing or visiting the embassy or consulate of the country you plan to visit (addresses of some embassies are at the end of this chapter). Your travel agent can apply for you, or you can use the services of a company that specializes in getting visas for travelers.

Many popular tourist destinations don't require visas — most western European countries, for example, and Caribbean nations. A list of countries requiring visas as well as passports is at the end of this chapter. But requirements change frequently, and to find out whether you need a tourist visa when you plan to take your trip, get a current copy of the State Department's pamphlet *Foreign Visa Requirements*. Send 50 cents to the Consumer Information Center, Pueblo, CO 81004.

After you write for an application, fill it out and send it in, along with your passport and whatever other documentation is asked for. Often one or more photos will be required. Some nations also want health certificates; others ask for translations of part of your passport into their own languages.

Send any application with your passport in it by registered mail.

There's a lot of passport politics. Some African nations won't let you in if your passport has a visa from South Africa. Though Israel doesn't require visas, some Arab countries will bar you from entry if you have an Israeli entrance or exit stamp on your passport. If you're visiting either country, get the passport agency to issue you two passports — one for Israel or South Africa, and the other for any other places you want to visit. Israeli authorities also will put your exit and entry stamps on a separate sheet of paper, if you ask for it.

If you think getting a visa sounds complicated, you're right. And time consuming, as well. If you're visiting several different countries that require visas, one way to simplify things is to contact a company in Washington or New York, where the embassies are, that specializes in getting visas for travelers. These companies also make it easy to get visas for travel groups. Their usual charge is $10 to $30 per visa — less for groups — plus the embassy fee and any expenses of postage or hand-delivery. Just send the company your passport, some photos and a list of visas you need. Some of them are:

In New York — Foreign Visa Service, 18 E. 93rd St., New York, NY 10028, ☎ 212/876-5890; Global Visa Service, 211 E. 43rd St., New York, NY 10017, ☎ (212/682-3895); Travel Agenda, Inc., 119 W. 57th St., Suite 1008, New York, NY 10019, ☎ 212/265-7887; Visa Center, Inc., 5407 Fifth Ave., New York, NY 10017, ☎ 212/986-0924; Visa Pioneers, Ltd., 25 E. 40th St., New York, NY 10016, ☎ 212/687-9477.

In Washington — Travisa, 2121 P. St. N.W., Washington, DC 20037, ☎ 202/328-1977, also branches in Detroit and Atlanta; Visa Expediters, Box 19444, Washington, DC 20036, ☎ 202/387-4789.

You can get a visa while you're traveling abroad — if you decide to add another country to your tour, for example. Wherever you are, apply to the representative of the country you want to visit, and be sure to have along the required photos and other paperwork.

If you're on a cruise, often you won't need a visa to go ashore in a country that otherwise requires them. Before you dock, the ship's purser is usually authorized to stamp your passport, identifying you as a passenger visiting only temporarily. Ask your travel agent before you go to the trouble of getting visas for these countries.

HEALTH CERTIFICATE

A few countries need certification that you're in good health and have had all the required shots.

Ask the local public health office (under "U.S. Government, Health & Human Services" in your phone book) for an International Certificate of Vaccination, and have your doctor fill in the appropriate page when you get your shot.

Carry with you a separate record of your shots, as well as other necessary health records discussed in Chapter 20.

PRESCRIPTIONS

One-third of Americans arrested abroad are held on drug charges. Remember, you're subject to local laws, not the U.S. Constitution, when you travel abroad.

To protect yourself from arrest if you're taking prescription drugs, carry a copy of your prescription along with a letter from your doctor explaining your need for the drug. Keep your prescriptions in their original containers.

VOUCHERS

Countries that maintain tight currency control may require you to buy a voucher before you leave the United States. It's a typical requirement for many eastern European nations.

Poland, for example requires you to buy vouchers worth $15 a day in zlotys for the length of your visit. You can spend the vouchers any way you want while you're there, but what you don't spend you have to leave behind. The requirements vary widely from country to country.

Each country will tell you about its currency requirements when it sends you a visa application.

CURRENCY REPORT

If you plan to leave the United States with more than $10,000 in any form — money orders, foreign or U.S. currency, traveler's checks, negotiable securities and the like — you have to report it to U.S. Customs when you leave and when you return.

File a Customs Form 4790 with the Customs Office at any port of entry or departure. You can get the form from most banks and travel agents.

INTERNATIONAL DRIVER'S LICENSE

Though your current state license is good in many places, there are advantages to getting an international driver's license if you plan to do any motoring — for one thing, it's written in several languages.

And some countries just don't recognize a U.S. driver's license.

You can get an international driver's license at any office of AAA, the National Automobile Club and the American Automobile Touring Alliance — whether or not you're a member.

TOURIST CARDS

Some countries that don't require you to get a visa will require you to carry a tourist card for identification.

Usually these are issued at the airline counter where you depart, or by immigration authorities when you get there. To avoid surprises, get the State Department's *Foreign Visa Requirements* bulletin, or ask your travel agent.

CERTIFICATES OF REGISTRATION

When you return to this country, U.S. Customs will charge you duty or taxes on any foreign-made item you're carrying — even your German camera, Japanese camcorder or Swiss watch — unless you can prove you had it when you went abroad.

Before you leave the United States, you can take any item that can be identified by serial number or other permanent marking to the nearest Customs Office for a Certificate of Registration.

If you don't live near a Customs Office, you can usually find one at the international airport or dock where you depart.

CERTIFICATES OF ORIGIN

It's illegal to sell ivory in the United States, but you can buy and sell antique scrimshawed ivory anywhere in the world.

You can't buy anything made from animals on the endangered species list in this country — but you can buy them abroad and bring them back in.

Some countries prohibit you from exporting their antiquities — but you can buy authentic-looking replicas.

Whenever there's any doubt whether it's legal in the United States to own the object you're buying abroad, get a Certificate of Origin from the seller attesting where the item came from and that its sale was legal.

SALES RECEIPTS

Whenever you buy anything abroad, keep the sales receipt. You'll need it to prove to U.S. Customs the value of the item when you declare it upon re-entry.

You also use sales receipts to claim any refunds for European Value Added Tax (VAT) you paid. In addition to the receipt, ask the sales clerk for an application to apply for the refund. See Chapter 17, Shopping, for details on claiming your VAT rebates.

YOUR ITINERARY

It's always wise to carry several copies of your travel itinerary.

One reason is that you need to register with the U.S. Embassy if you're planning to stay in a country more than a month. They'll ask for a copy of your itinerary so they can find you in an emergency.

You also need to register with an embassy — and provide an itinerary — if you're going to an Eastern Bloc country, a country where there's no U.S. representation or one with an unstable political climate.

Some foreign immigration officials may also ask for your itinerary as proof of where you intend to travel in their countries.

Carry your papers in two safe places — on your body, in your hand-luggage or in your clothing bags. But, store only duplicate items and records — your list of travelers check numbers, for instance — in your luggage. You can carry critical papers that you'll need often — your passport, for example — in a passport wallet strapped to your body or in an inside pocket.

IN SUMMARY:

— Start early to get your travel papers in order.
— Ask your travel agent to help you get visas.
— Make sure you know paperwork requirements for every country you're visiting.

★ ★ ★
Travel Tool
★ ★ ★

A PAPERWORK CHECKLIST

Wherever you go, get started early collecting the required papers. Find out whether you'll need to bring your:

- Passport
- Visa
- Tourist Card
- Currency Vouchers
- Health or Vaccination Certificate
- Other needed health records
- Drug prescriptions and physicians' letter of explanation
- Physician's phone number
- International Driver's License
- Certificates of Registration for foreign-made personal possessions
- U.S. Currency Report
- Copies of your itinerary
- Photocopy of your passport's data page
- Record of traveler's-check numbers
- Record of credit-card numbers
- Record of travel agent's phone number, or emergency numbers abroad
- Record of U.S. consulate addresses and phone numbers.

★ ★ ★
Travel Tool
★ ★ ★

COUNTRIES REQUIRING VISAS

Here are countries requiring visas for entry, as well as U.S. passports, as reported in the latest U.S. State Department Bureau of Consular Affairs bulletin, *Foreign Visa Requirements*. Remember that these requirements change frequently, and you should check with the embassy or consulate of the country you want to visit for latest requirements.

- Afghanistan
- Albania
- Algeria
- Andorra
- Angola
- Argentina
- Australia
- Bahrain
- Benin
- Bhutan
- Brazil
- Brunei
- Bulgaria
- Burkina Faso
- Burma
- Burundi
- Cameroon
- Cape Verde
- Central African Republic
- Chad
- China
- Colombia
- Comoros Island
- Congo
- Cuba
- Czechoslovakia
- Dahomey
- Djibouti
- East Germany

- Egypt
- El Salvador
- Equatorial Guinea
- Estonia
- Ethiopia
- Fuji
- France
- French Guiana
- French West Indies (at port of entry)
- Gabon
- Gambia
- Ghana
- Guadeloupe
- Guatemala
- Guinea-Bissau
- Guyana
- Honduras
- Hungary
- India
- Iran
- Iraq
- Ivory Coast
- Jordan
- Kampuchea
- Kenya
- Kiribati
- Kuwait
- Laos
- Latvia

- Lebanon
- Liberia
- Libya
- Lithuania
- Macau
- Madagascar
- Mali
- Martinique
- Mauritania
- Mayotte Island
- Miquelon
- Monaco
- Mongolia
- Mozambique
- Nauru
- Nepal
- New Caledonia
- Niger
- Nigeria
- North Korea
- Oman
- Pakistan
- Panama
- Poland
- Qatar
- Reunion
- Romania
- Russia
- Rwanda
- St. Barthelemy

- St. Pierre
- Sao Tome and Principe
- Saudi Arabia
- Senegal
- Sierra Leone
- Somali
- South Africa
- South Korea

- Sudan
- Suriname
- Syria
- Tahiti
- Taiwan
- Tanzania
- Tuvalu
- Uganda

- United Arab Emirates
- Venezuela
- Vietnam
- Yemen, North and South
- Yugoslavia
- Zaire

★ ★ ★
Travel Tool
★ ★ ★

HOW TO GET A VISA

Here's how to find out visa requirements for some popular tourist destinations:

Argentina
Argentine Embassy, 1600 New Hampshire Ave., Washington DC 20009.
☎ 202/939-6400.
Also consulates in Baltimore, Chicago, Houston, Los Angeles, Miami, New Orleans, New York, San Francisco, Puerto Rico.

Australia
Australian Embassy, 1601 Massachusetts Ave. N.W., Washington, DC 20036.
☎ 202/797-3000.
Also consulates general in San Francisco, New York, Chicago, Honolulu, Los Angeles, Houston.

Brazil
Brazilian Embassy, 3006 Massachusetts Ave. N.W., Washington, DC 20008.
☎ 202/745-2700.

China
Chinese Embassy, 2300 Connecticut Ave. N.W., Washington, DC 20008.
☎ 202/328-2500.
Also consulates general in San Francisco, Houston, New York.

Egypt
Egyptian Consulate, 2300 Decatur Place, Washington, DC 20008.
☎ 202/234-3903.
Also consulates in Chicago, Houston, San Francisco, New York.

France
French Consulate, 4101 Reservoir Rd., Washington, DC 20002.
☎ 202/944-6200
Also consulates in Boston, Chicago, Detroit, Houston, Los Angeles, Miami, New York, New Orleans, Puerto Rico, San Francisco.

East Germany
Embassy of the GDR, 1717 Massachusetts Ave. N.W., Washington, DC 20036.
☎ 202/232-3134.

Hungary
Hungarian Embassy, 3910 Shoemaker St. N.W, Washington, DC 20008.
☎ 202/362-6730.
Also consulate-general in New York.

India
Indian Embassy, Washington, DC 20008.
☎ 202/939-9839.
Also consulates in New York, Chicago, San Francisco.

Japan
Japanese Embassy, 2502 Massachusetts Ave., Washington, DC 20008.
☎ 202/939-6700.

Kenya
Kenya Embassy, 2249 K St. N.W., Washington, DC 20008.
☎ 202/387-6101.
Also tourist offices in New York, Beverly Hills, Calif.

Poland
Polish Embassy, 2224 Wyoming Ave. N.W., Washington, DC 20008.
☎ 202/234-3800.
Also consulates general in Chicago, New York.

South Africa
Republic of South Africa Embassy, 3051 Massachusetts Ave. N.W., Washington, DC 20008.
☎ 202/232-4400
Also consulates-general in New York, Beverly Hills, Houston, Chicago.

South Korea
South Korean Embassy, 2600 Virginia Ave. N.W., Suite 200, Watergate Building, Washington, DC 20037.
☎ 202/939-5600.

Taiwan
Coordination Council for North American Affairs, 4201 Wisconsin Ave. N.W., Washington, DC 20016.
☎ 202/895-1800
Additional offices in Atlanta, Boston, Chicago, Honolulu, Houston, Kansas City, Los Angeles, New York, San Francisco, Seattle.

Yugoslavia
Yugoslav Embassy, 9410 California St. N.W., Washington, DC 20008.
☎ 202/462-6566.

Travel Tool

★ ★ ★

WHERE YOU CAN GO WITHOUT A PASSPORT

Here are nations not requiring U.S. passports or visas for entry, as reported in the most recent *Foreign Visa Requirements* from the U.S. State Department's Bureau of Consular Affairs. Remember that most of these nations, however, do require some proof of U.S. citizenship.

- Anguilla
- Antigua
- Aruba
- Bahamas
- Barbuda
- Barbados
- Bermuda
- Bonaire
- Cayman Islands
- Canada
- Curacao
- Dominica
- Haiti
- Marshall Islands
- Mexico
- Micronesia
- Montserrat
- Norfolk Island
- Palau
- Panama
- Saba
- Statia
- St .Kitts and Nevis
- St. Lucia
- St. Martin/Maarten
- St. Vincent/Grenadines
- Turks and Caicos
- Virgin Islands

CHAPTER 8

COUNTDOWN TO V-(FOR VACATION) DAY

| For Every Packing Problem, There's a Solution |

When your travels take you from a 25-below-zero Minneapolis morning to an 85-above Acapulco afternoon, how do you plan for it without freezing, sweltering or hauling your entire closet on your back?

It isn't easy, but for every travel-packing problem, there is a solution.

We have friends from the Midwest who make the journey to the sun every winter. Some are snowbirds, and they do carry their closets on their backs — in their vans and motorhomes. Others, who just want a two-week respite from the cold, need to turn on the creative energy to pack light.

One Minnesota friend refuses to cope with her overcoat in the Bahamas and adds a thermal layer. She wears a thermal shirt under her blouse, then dresses as if she were walking to the store on a cool fall evening by adding either a raincoat, light jacket or sweater and scarf. As the plane wings its way south, she moves into the restroom where she takes the thermal shirt off and puts it in her carry-on bag. When she flies home, she reverses the process. She keeps warm without needing a bulky coat. Her brainpower makes it easy on her back.

WEATHER WATCH

This is the stage of travel planning that we think of as "milling about." We find it far better to make lists and discard them, and to pack and unpack in our minds than to reach our destination too bogged down with baggage to move, or missing the one thing we really needed — like a tennis racquet if we're seeded in a tournament.

Our travel countdown requires learning something about the weather and terrain where we're heading. We check such information sources as the National Weather Service (listed in your phone book under U.S. Commerce, Dept. of, National Weather Service), our daily newspaper, the Weather Channel, and travel periodicals such as *Travel and Leisure*. Bookstores carry special guides that describe special clothing needs for different cities. For example, *Weather Travelpack* offers suggestions on what to pack for 50 different U.S. cities for every month of the year. Others cover cities in Europe and Latin America. If your bookstore doesn't carry them, write Weather Trends International Ltd., 156 Fifth Ave., New York, NY 10010.

And while we are learning about an area in general, we look for specific data like the average high temperature, average low temperature, average rainfall or snowfall, number of rain days during the month of our stay, average humidity and elevation. These numbers will tell us what kind of coat to pack, whether to carry along an umbrella or boots, whether our clothes should be made of predominantly natural fibers and whether the temperature will begin to drop when the sun goes to bed.

We also analyze our itinerary for details about the facilities available and the activities planned. Even if we're going to Chicago in December, we'd hate to leave our swimsuits at home, only to find that the hotel has an indoor pool and spa. Nor do we want to lug our golf clubs along — even to a resort — if there's no time allotted to play. And we don't want to have to head for the hotel cafeteria for a sandwich when the schedule calls for dinner with the governor — just because we brought nothing but casual clothes.

As one Alaska cruise director said, the advice to "dress casual" doesn't always help much. "Does casual mean sneakers and sweats, or women in country-club dresses and men in blazers with gray flannel slacks?"

MAKING LISTS

One of our favorite countdown techniques is to make a list of days, divided into thirds. Then we begin to fill in known planned activities and to match clothes to the activities. This kind of a list does double duty. Not only does it guarantee that we'll have just enough of the right clothes for each occasion, but it also serves as an inventory of what we're taking. That way, if our luggage should be lost or stolen, we have an itemized list for insurance purposes. For example:

Monday morning: on plane — He: slacks, sportshirt, blazer, loafers. She: pant suit, blouse, flats.

Monday afternoon: check-in, orientation — He: same as plane. She: same as plane.

Monday evening: VIP reception, dinner — He: dress shirt, blue suit, tie. She: navy cocktail dress, heels.

Tuesday morning: city bus tour — He: khakis, sport shirt, jacket, walking shoes. She: slacks, blouse, jacket, walking shoes.

Tuesday afternoon: marketplace excursion — He: same as morning. She: same as morning.

Tuesday evening: barbecue, country western music — He: same as morning, change shirt and shoes. She: same as morning, change blouse and shoes.

We fill in this daily list as completely as possible for the entire trip. Then by using two rules of thumb, we begin to eliminate items.

One rule is to admit that we are dressing for appropriateness and comfort, not for a fashion magazine, nor to impress our fellow travelers. That will help us toss out at least a few items.

The second rule is to limit clothing to two basic colors. A reader of *Friendly Exchange* magazine put it this way: "To coordinate your clothes, take a print blouse and match two of the colors in it with slacks or skirts. A man could do the same with a tie. The rule is, take a print and match it twice and you're always sure to look very nice. This rule will force us to think about what goes with what. The result is that more items are put back into the closet."

After the daily list, we make a separate list of what we call "extras." The extras will be different, depending on the trip and the person, but ours generally include accessories, outerwear, underwear, shoes (at least two pairs), sporting equipment, cameras, money (see chapter 6, Money Matters), security items (see chapter 21, Protecting Yourself), medicines (see chapter 20, To Your Health), and, especially, desirable creature comforts.

There's a lot to be said for creature comforts. While we're strong believers in packing light, we also advocate the joy of travel. And if you're a person who gets cranky when you get hungry, by all means pack some of your favorite snacks or you may not have much joy on your journey. If your skin craves a specific kind of lotion or moisturizer, take along enough for the entire trip; you don't want to waste hours trying to find a specific brand. If you can't sleep without your teddy, tuck him into your case.

PUTTING THE RIGHT FOOT FORWARD

Among the most important things you'll pack will be shoes. They do add weight and bulk. On the other hand, a poor choice of shoes could limit your ability to do everything you planned.

Plan to pack at least two pairs of comfortable walking shoes and alternate wearing them. Do not buy and take new or untried shoes on a trip.

Men should take an additional pair of dressy loafers or casual oxfords for use whenever you're not wearing your walking shoes. Women need an extra pair of super-comfortable flats and a pair of dress heels. If you're heading into wet or snowy country, you may swap a light pair of flat-heeled boots for the flat shoes. They offer protection from the weather and will wear nicely with slacks, casual skirts and the like. We each carry walking shoes — and we mean special athletic shoes designed for walking. They are built for maximum support and comfort and will go almost anywhere in daylight hours. They can also double for a quick trip to the beach.

If walking shoes are new to you, head for your nearest sporting goods store and try on a pair or two. Make sure you ask for walking shoes, because shoes made for tennis or aerobics or even running are built differently.

When you shop, wear the same kind of socks you plan to wear with the shoes and try walking on concrete — not on the store's rug. The shoes should feel good the first time you put them on. Look for a shoe that keeps your heel snug, while giving your toes plenty of room to spread out. Make sure the shoe's arch support matches the contours of your feet's arches. Look for a sole made of durable material with a textured tread that will retain traction on slippery surfaces. Buy them and wear them for a couple of weeks before taking them on a trip.

PACKING IT IN

There are two basic schools of thought when it comes to packing. One is to wait until the day before the trip, then put as much into the suitcase as it will hold and pray that you have everything you need for the journey. A friend who packs this way on a regular basis wound up in Mexico with the sports shirts he purchased for the occasion at home in his dresser drawer. Another time, he found himself in San Francisco without any socks. While that kind of packing may do something for the economy you're visiting, it also means you'll spend some unexpected time shopping.

The second school of thought is to set out everything you want to take, and pack half of it. You may still wind up carrying along more than you need.

We don't subscribe to either school, since we've developed a system that works for us trip after trip. It's based on the list we described earlier.

What did take some trial and error, however, was finding the right suitcase. Our first choice was one enormous suitcase for each of us — big enough to put an old-fashioned steamer trunk to shame. Then we found ourselves pinned to a train station in Venice once because we could not find a porter and we could not carry our own bags. That's when we began looking for alternatives.

Now we have a totally mismatched set of luggage that works no matter how long or short the trip. Our choices:

For the traveling lady: two flat pullmans, one a 21-incher, the other a 23-incher. The small one is used for trips of five days or less; the larger for up to two weeks. If the journey is 100 percent casual — meaning just slacks, sweatshirts and the like, substitute a soft-sided duffel.

For the traveling gentleman: a one-suiter fold-up garment bag that fits under an airline seat for trips of five days or less. For longer journeys, it's a floppy duffel that seems to expand to hold almost as much as a steamer trunk.

None of this luggage is expensive. All the bags are sturdy without being heavy. All are water-resistant. All have working locks.

Since the kind of bag you choose is determined by the kinds of clothing you need to carry with you, the decision is a very personal one. But there's lots of help available. For example, study the most current *Consumer Reports* evaluation of luggage. To find it, ask your local reference librarian. Such a survey will describe important questions to ask or criteria to use in making your own decision. Write for literature. Samsonite offers a booklet, *Getting a Handle on Luggage,* that's available by writing to 11200 E. 45th Ave., Denver, CO 80239. The DuPont Company offers *How To Pack Soft-Sided Luggage* if you send a stamped, addressed business-size envelope to the Fibers Department, Laurel Run Building, P.O. Box 80705, Wilmington, DE 19890-0705. These booklets also offer great ideas for packing efficiently and easily.

After reading, head for your nearest luggage store. Look at bags of the same size created by different manufacturers. Look at the way they're made. Are the seams stitched straight, and are the threads unbroken? Does the material have a smooth finish or will it snag your clothes? Do the zippers and locks work smoothly and easily? Are the handles and straps comfortable, well anchored and strong enough to carry the suitcase loaded? Are the screws or rivets properly seated? Are the pockets and dividers really useful? If it's a garment bag, does the clothing bar have a means to lock in or alternate hangers?

Imagine the items you'll carry in the bag. Is there room for the cosmetic or toiletries kit you use? Is the bag deep enough to allow you to pack shoes? Is there a way to pack suits or long dresses in the space available?

Finally, ask if the bag can be returned. Take your choice home and pack it with your usual quantity of clothing. Try carrying the full bag around your living room for a few minutes. If it doesn't work, take the unused, undamaged bag back to the store and try a different one.

WHAT TO PACK

Show us two different travel books, and we'll show you two different "perfect" travel wardrobes. For the most part, the lists are all-purpose since they don't take into consideration activities, personal interests, weather, local customs and such.

We have found that most trips can be handled with some old reliables. The traveling lady, for example, almost always takes a three-piece suit — jacket, skirt and slacks — in a basic color. Then she'll add a second, compatibly colored jacket, a second pair of slacks and a variety of tops including a fancy, jeweled or frilly one. With a dressy dress, if it's needed, and a pair of washable slacks and raincoat, this group of clothes will cover most needs for a week or more unless we're in a country where the combination of women and pants is considered poor manners. Then swap the slacks for skirts.

The traveling gentleman usually takes a suit, compatible blazer and slacks, a couple of pairs of washable khakis and a variety of shirts.

Where the lists can really help, however, is with the accessories or options, those "I-wish-I'd-thought-of-that" travel extras. Here are some things we find handy:

• Warmup suit. Especially good for a cruise. It can be used for the exercise classes, for lounging or walking. And it doesn't wrinkle.

• Golf-style windbreaker jacket. The kind you can fit into a purse or pocket, the kind with a hood folded into its collar. It's great for places where the temperature drops after dark, or where there are surprise showers.

• Head covering. The most adaptable one we've seen is a fabric fold-up hat that protects from either sun or cold. Somes call it a "bucket hat," others simply call it a rain hat.

• Binoculars. If you're going where the wildlife watching is good (like an Alaska Inside Passage cruise), or if your itinerary includes theatrical events.

• Electrical converters, if needed. Ask your travel agent.

• Bottle opener, corkscrew and so on. Many of our friends carry a Swiss Army knife with all the attachments. But be sure to carry it in your checked suitcase, not on your person. It is, after all, a weapon.

• Sponge or washcloth and small soap bar.
• Several sizes of plastic bags to use for dirty clothes, wet swimsuits and the like.
• Small notebook or diary to record trip details, names and addresses.
• Language phrase book, maps, guidebooks.
• Sewing kit including safety pins and small scissors.
• Travel alarm clock.
• Packets of tissues and/or moist towelettes.
• Gifts for hosts such as music cassettes, seed packets, charms from our hometown.
• Folding umbrella.
• Pre-addressed labels to use to send gifts or cards home, or to send film for processing.
• Extra luggage keys.
• Surgical face mask if you have breathing problems and air pollution is a possibility.
• Medical kit with duplicate prescriptions, doctor's phone number, vaccination certificates and the like (see chapter 20, To Your Health, for itemized list).
• Camera equipment and supplies, including extra batteries and film, as well as mail-in film-processing envelopes.
• Laundry detergent concentrate, flat sink stopper and pincher clothespins.
• Hair-care supplies including shower cap.
• Pocket calculator for figuring exchange rates.
• Time-killers such as books, playing cards, travel-size version of games like backgammon or Scrabble.
• Athletic equipment. If a swimsuit is your main athletic equipment, include a coverup that doubles as a robe, and beach sandals.
• Copies of your itinerary with dates, flight numbers, phone numbers, reservation confirmations — one to carry, one to keep inside your suitcase.
• Extra bag that folds flat to be used to carry home your shopping finds.

TAKING IT WITH YOU

Pack as if you plan to lose your luggage.

The most important bag of all is the carry-on, the one you keep with you at all times. Carefully planned, the carry-on should be able to see you through at least 36 hours without your bigger bag. Keep these items with you:
- Medicines, eyeglasses, prescriptions.
- Passport, travel documents, money, vital numbers.
- Night clothes.
- Change of clothing such as underwear and blouse or shirt and shoes.
- Airport entertainment items.
- Itinerary and inventory.
- Snacks that can get you through an unexpected flight delay. Some of our choices include oatmeal cookies or packages of raisins.

IN SUMMARY:

— Before you pack, check the weather where you're going.
— Match clothes to your expected activities.
— Do not take new shoes on a trip.
— Don't pack a bag bigger than you can carry yourself.
— Pack as if you plan to lose your bags.

★ ★ ★
Travel Tool
★ ★ ★

WEATHER AROUND THE WORLD

Here are seasonal high and low temperatures for cities around the world, along with the number of days per month of precipitation — rain or snow. Use this is a guide to selecting what clothes to take.

LOCATION	JAN	FEB	MAR	APR	MAY	JUN	JUL	AUG	SEP	OCT	NOV	DEC	
Acapulco	88	88	88	88	90	90	91	91	90	90	90	88	HI TEMP
	72	72	72	73	77	77	77	77	77	77	75	75	LO TEMP
	0	8	0	2	2	13	15	14	16	8	2	1	DAYS PRECIP.
Athens	54	57	61	67	77	86	90	91	84	74	66	59	HI TEMP
	42	45	46	52	61	68	72	73	66	60	54	46	LO TEMP
	7	6	5	3	3	2	1	1	2	4	6	7	DAYS PRECIP.

LOCATION	JAN	FEB	MAR	APR	MAY	JUN	JUL	AUG	SEP	OCT	NOV	DEC	
Beijing	33	42	53	70	80	88	89	86	78	66	50	40	HI TEMP
	16	21	32	44	56	65	72	70	57	44	30	20	LO TEMP
	2	2	2	3	5	7	15	11	8	2	1	2	DAYS PRECIP.
Cairo	65	69	75	88	91	95	96	95	90	86	78	68	HI TEMP
	47	48	52	57	63	68	70	71	68	65	58	50	LO TEMP
	1	1	1	0	0	0	0	0	0	0	1	1	DAYS PRECIP.
Hong	64	62	66	75	82	84	87	88	84	81	74	68	HI TEMP
Kong	56	56	60	67	74	78	78	78	77	73	65	59	LO TEMP
	4	5	7	8	13	18	17	15	12	6	2	3	DAYS PRECIP.
Jeru-	56	56	65	74	81	85	88	88	85	81	70	59	HI TEMP
salem	41	43	47	50	58	61	63	65	63	59	54	45	LO TEMP
	8	8	5	3	0	0	0	0	0	1	5	6	DAYS PRECIP.
London	44	47	49	56	63	68	73	72	65	58	49	47	HI TEMP
	35	36	38	40	47	52	55	54	50	44	40	38	LO TEMP
	6	5	5	5	5	6	6	13	6	7	6	7	DAYS PRECIP.
Madrid	47	52	59	64	70	81	87	86	77	66	55	48	HI TEMP
	33	36	41	44	50	59	62	63	57	48	41	36	LO TEMP
	8	87	10	9	10	5	2	3	6	8	9	11	DAYS PRECIP.
Montreal	21	25	36	50	65	74	78	77	68	54	42	27	HI TEMP
	6	12	23	33	48	58	61	58	53	40	32	16	LO TEMP
	17	15	13	13	13	12	13	12	12	12	15	17	DAYS PRECIP.
Moscow	212	22	322	47	67	70	76	72	61	46	36	23	HI TEMP
	9	7	18	311	47	52	55	54	45	34	27	14	LO TEMP
	18	15	15	13	13	12	15	14	13	20	15	23	DAYS PRECIP.
Munich	34	38	49	58	65	70	74	74	68	56	45	36	HI TEMP
	26	23	31	38	45	52	56	54	49	40	32	25	LO TEMP
	16	16	133	15	15	17	16	16	13	13	15	15	DAYS PRECIP.
Nassau	77	77	79	81	85	88	88	90	88	85	81	79	HI TEMP
	65	65	67	69	72	74	75	76	76	73	70	67	LO TEMP
	6	5	5	6	9	12	14	14	15	13	9	6	DAYS PRECIP.
Paris	42	45	54	60	68	73	76	75	70	59	50	45	HI TEMP
	32	34	39	41	50	55	55	57	54	44	41	36	LO TEMP
	17	14	12	13	12	12	12	13	13	13	15	16	DAYS PRECIP.
Rio de	84	85	83	80	77	76	75	76	75	77	79	82	HI TEMP
Janeiro	73	73	72	69	66	64	63	64	65	66	68	71	LO TEMP
	13	11	12	10	10	7	7	7	11	13	13	14	DAYS PRECIP.
Rome	54	55	59	68	73	82	88	86	79	73	61	55	HI TEMP
	39	41	45	46	55	63	64	66	63	53	48	43	LO TEMP
	8	9	8	6	5	4	1	2	5	8	11	10	DAYS PRECIP.
Stockholm	30	30	37	46	57	66	72	68	59	48	41	36	HI TEMP
	23	23	25	34	43	52	57	55	48	41	34	28	LO TEMP
	16	14	10	11	11	13	13	14	14	15	16	17	DAYS PRECIP.
Sydney	78	79	76	71	67	61	60	63	67	71	74	77	HI TEMP
	65	65	63	58	52	49	46	48	52	56	61	63	LO TEMP
	14	13	14	14	13	12	12	11	12	12	12	13	DAYS PRECIP.
Tokyo	47	48	53	63	72	75	83	86	78	69	60	51	HI TEMP
	29	30	35	46	53	62	70	72	66	55	42	33	LO TEMP
	5	6	10	10	10	12	10	9	12	11	7	5	DAYS PRECIP.
Vancouver	41	45	48	58	60	65	74	71	65	57	48	43	HI TEMP
	32	36	37	40	47	52	54	55	52	44	39	35	LO TEMP
	20	16	17	14	10	9	6	9	10	16	19	22	DAYS PRECIP.
Venice	43	46	54	63	70	77	81	81	75	66	54	46	HI TEMP
	34	36	41	50	57	63	66	64	61	52	45	37	LO TEMP
	6	6	7	9	8	8	7	7	5	7	9	8	DAYS PRECIP.

★ ★ ★
Travel Tool
★ ★ ★

CLIMATE IN THE U. S.

Here are seasonal high and low temperatures for U.S. cities, along with the number of days per month of precipitation — rain or snow.

LOCATION	JAN	FEB	MAR	APR	MAY	JUN	JUL	AUG	SEP	OCT	NOV	DEC	
Anchorage	22	25	31	43	55	62	65	63	55	41	27	20	HI TEMP
	7	9	14	27	38	47	50	49	40	27	14	6	LO TEMP
	3	3	2	2	1	4	7	7	6	5	3	3	DAYS PRECIP.
Chicago	31	34	45	59	70	79	83	82	75	66	48	35	HI TEMP
	15	18	27	38	47	57	61	60	52	42	30	19	LO TEMP
	11	11	13	13	11	10	10	9	10	10	10	11	DAYS PRECIP.
Honolulu	79	79	80	81	84	86	87	87	87	86	83	80	HI TEMP
	65	65	66	68	70	72	73	74	73	72	70	67	LO TEMP
	10	10	9	9	7	6	8	7	7	9	9	10	DAYS PRECIP.
Las Vegas	60	66	71	80	89	98	102	102	95	84	71	60	HI TEMP
	28	33	39	44	51	60	68	66	57	46	35	30	LO TEMP
	1	1	1	1	1	0	1	1	1	1	1	1	DAYS PRECIP.
Los Angeles	67	68	69	71	73	77	83	84	83	78	73	68	HI TEMP
	47	49	50	53	56	60	68	66	57	46	35	30	LO TEMP
	6	5	6	4	1	1	0	1	1	2	3	5	DAYS PRECIP.
Miami	76	77	80	83	85	88	89	90	88	85	80	77	HI TEMP
	59	59	63	67	71	74	67	76	75	71	65	60	LO TEMP
	7	6	5	6	11	15	16	17	17	15	8	7	DAYS PRECIP.
New York	39	40	48	61	71	81	85	83	77	67	54	41	HI TEMP
	26	27	34	44	53	63	68	66	60	51	41	30	LO TEMP
	11	10	12	11	11	10	10	10	8	8	9	10	DAYS PRECIP.
San Francisco	56	59	60	61	63	65	64	65	69	68	63	57	HI TEMP
	46	48	49	49	51	53	53	54	56	55	52	47	LO TEMP
	11	10	10	6	3	1	1	1	1	4	8	10	DAYS PRECIP.
Washington D.C.	44	46	55	67	77	85	88	87	80	70	57	45	HI TEMP
	28	29	35	46	56	65	69	68	61	51	39	30	LO TEMP
	11	9	11	10	11	9	10	9	8	7	8	9	DAYS PRECIP.

Climate data is provided by

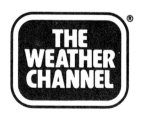

NOTES

CHAPTER 9

COVERING THE HOME FRONT

Who'll Watch the House While You're Away?

Hi, said the bright voice on the telephone answering machine, "Bill and Mary Jones are on a well-deserved cruise in the Caribbean. Just leave a message, and we'll return your call when we get back on September first."

It should have been no surprise to the Joneses that they returned to an empty house, picked clean by thieves.

Ninety percent of people recording their own answering machine messages announce that, "We're not home right now," according to telephone company estimates, and many of those also tell thieves exactly how much time they'll have to knock over the place.

Instead of broadcasting their absence, the Joneses should have left an innocuous message that said something like:

"Hi. You have reached 123-4567. Please leave your message at the sound of the tone." Without even a family name.

The Joneses wouldn't have missed a single call. And they wouldn't be missing their furniture.

A GOING-AWAY ROUTINE

The telephone-answering-machine message is just one of the major clues that modern professional thieves use to plan their workdays. The grass grows long, the papers and mail pile up, the lights stay off — those are other clues thieves use.

It's no fun coming home from a trip to find burglars have used the clues you left behind to do their work while you've been at play. So it's worth your time to develop a checklist for your peace of mind and security.

We have regular routines — depending on whether the trip is going to be a long weekend, a few weeks or longer. For example, the captain sets the lights and locks and handles the mail and newspapers; the first mate cleans the Fridge, cares for the yard and organizes the cleaning help. It's become so automatic that we seldom use a checklist for the short trips anymore.

The longer journeys are a different story. We make lists well in advance. Routines for all of our trips evolved from studying our living patterns and making sure that our house would look lived-in while we were on the road. Here are some ways to do that:

THE NEIGHBORHOOD PLAN

Many neighborhoods work together; you tell one neighbor when you'll be gone and that neighbor collects your mail and newspapers, calls the police if something looks awry, mows and waters your yard (or shovels your walk), parks a car in your driveway periodically, puts a trash barrel out and does any other tasks necessary to make your house look lived-in and looked-out for. When that neighbor travels, you return the favor.

HOUSESITTERS

If you want more attention or if you're going to be gone for a longer time, you may want to hire a housesitter — either someone who lives in your home full time while you're away, or a person who will stop by one or two times a day to handle needed miscellaneous tasks.

If you hire a housesitter, start interviewing early, since professional sitters are booked well in advance. Professionals can be found in newspaper classified sections or telephone-book Yellow Pages under "Sitting Services."

Professionals such as those supplied by Home Sitting Services, a franchise located in more than 85 cities, are bonded and insured and cost $22 to $72 a day, depending on the going rates in your area. Sitters under contract to Home Sitting Services are generally seniors in good health — people like you who want the opportunity to be useful and independent — who agree to stay your home 22 of every 24 hours. They are not there to do maintenance or cleaning work, but they do agree to clean up after themselves.

If you're willing to work with amateurs, your fellow retirees make great housesitters. Contact a senior-citizens center or group in your area. Another source of sitters is colleges; they often have visiting staff members or teachers on sabbatical who need temporary housing; or try a college placement office for students needing work.

If you are considering a professional sitting service, first contact your Better Business Bureau and police department to see if there have been any complaints filed against the company. And contact your own attorney to set up any special powers-of-attorney that may be needed — such as a medical power-of-attorney for your pet.

If you're interviewing sitters, be prepared with questions that are important to you, such as:

How much time will they spend in the home?

Do they have references?

Are they comfortable with pets?

And so on until you are satisfied. Ask each candidate the same questions and give each the same information to work with.

When it comes time to leave on your trip, have the sitter come a couple of hours before your departure. Walk the sitter through the house with your housebook in hand. Leave adequate time for questions.

THE HOUSEBOOK

Whether it's a neighbor or a hired sitter looking after the house, you should create a housebook: a catalogue of information and idiosyncrasies about your house and belongings — including your car — that a temporary resident would need to know. Include information about service people such as gardeners and plumbers who can be relied on in emergencies, operating manuals for the major appliances, names and phone numbers of insurance companies with policies, plant-watering routines, car-registration data and the like. No book will be the same for every house, but a worksheet to get you started is at the end of this chapter.

PROTECTING IT YOURSELF

If you're going to trust to your own abilities to safeguard your home, start by calling your local police department. Some police departments will survey your home and tell you about ineffective security devices or locks you may be using. But even if they can't analyze your safety steps, most police departments want to know if you're going to be gone so they can check on your home periodically. Give the police a phone number and address where you can be reached if needed in an emergency.

In addition, prepare your home by:

• Doing a thorough yard cleanup; pruning back bushes from windows and doors.

• Updating your home inventory and putting it in a safe place.

• Checking windows and doors for needed repairs and locks, and fixing them; locking all doors when you leave and immobilizing sliding doors and windows, preferably with key-operated locks.

• Putting small valuables in your safety deposit box; etching identification on larger items.

• Checking and updating important documents such as your insurance, power-of-attorney and will.

•Hooking up radios and lamps to variable timers and making sure all lights — inside and out — attached to timers have fresh bulbs.

• Giving one trustworthy neighbor or relative your itinerary. That same person can keep a duplicate list of numbers such as passports, travelers checks, and credit cards in case you need them. Your trusted friend should also be given a house key and the name of a person — such as your attorney — to call in case of an emergency at your home or if you become sick or die.

• Paying all the bills you can in advance.

• Making decisions about how mail will be handled; putting your mail on vacation hold at the post office or contracting with a mail-forwarding service. If you want to receive mail as you travel, you may want it sent to your hotel general delivery in cities you will visit. American Express now limits its mail service to credit-card or traveler's-check customers, and it is not available in all cities.

- Leaving your lawn sprinklers on a timer or continuing your normal yard-care and pool-care services.
- Cleaning out your refrigerator.
- Discussing vacation options about both service and bills with your utility companies. They can also advise you on the best settings for thermostats to prevent problems with frozen pipes and such.
- Canceling services such as newspapers or other deliveries.
- Having a great time!

IN SUMMARY:

— Set up a going-away routine, complete with checklist.
— Ask a neighbor or a paid house-sitter to watch over the house while you're gone.
— Develop a housebook to help others take care of the place.
— Don't invite thieves in with your phone answering machine.

★ ★ ★
Travel Tool
★ ★ ★

HOW TO CREATE A HOUSEBOOK

Start with a large yellow tablet that you keep close at hand for a week or so. Jot down everything as you think of it about your home, contents, service personnel, yard, pets, car and neighborhood. You'll be surprised how much detail there is involved in running your home. After you've made your notes, sort them into categories and fill in details such as phone numbers, warranties and the like. When you've finished, you'll have a record you can add to or update for each trip. Here are some subjects to consider when making your first housebook:

Car — Registration, insurance, service center.

Service Personnel — Large appliances, plumbing, electrical, swimming pool/spa, yard, insurance agent, garage door, housecleaner, alarm system.

Utilities — Water, gas, electric (including where the water meter, cutoff valve and fuse boxes are located), phone emergency services — police, fire, doctor, hospital, ambulance, veterinarian.

Neighbors and Neighborhood — Names with addresses and phone numbers, trash pickup days and times; post office location.

Large Appliances — Warranties, operating manuals and idiosyncrasies.

Telephone System — Including answering machine and how it works.

Itinerary — Where you will be daily, with addresses and phone numbers and any other duplicate numbers you want access to by long distance phone.

Pets — Where the animals sleep, what they eat, their distinctive habits, medication or ailments.

Legal Matters — Your family attorney, location of will, pet power of attorney.

No-Nos — An itemized list of things not to be used.

Mail Instructions — How you want your mail handled and what should be forwarded.

Landscaping and Plants — Care and watering schedule.

Periodicals — Newspapers and magazines subscribed to.

Bills to be Paid — Along with a small amount of money to handle a cash-only emergency repair, instructions on what to do with bills received.

Oddities — The light switch that controls the television set or the hidden steering-wheel lock on your car. The kinds of things only an insider would know.

II

WAYS TO GO

You can drive, fly or cruise to the vacation of your dreams.

CHAPTER 10

BY AUTOMOBILE

When You're in Your Car, the Trip Belongs to You

There is no way to travel that gives 49ers-plus more freedom than going by automobile.

You can set your own pace — stop by the roadside to look at the scenery when you want, pull in for coffee or a pit stop whenever you feel the need, get up and drive as early as you want, or stop for the day whenever you get tired. You're bound only by your own timetable.

You can drive an auto down narrow alleys and up twisting mountain roads you'd never think of navigating with an RV, make your way in to remote sites that a motorcoach wouldn't attempt.

And the automobile puts you closer to the people and the countryside than any other means of travel except, perhaps, foot or horseback. You can get off the freeway onto narrow byways, drive into little towns and villages you'd never see on a tour, spend an extra night at a country inn you enjoy, take in a carnival or a festival.

In your car, the trip is all yours.

JOINING AN AUTO CLUB

For the $30 to $50 it costs, joining an auto club can be a bargain if you're planning a long motor trip.

We joined the American Automobile Association (AAA) just before we took a winter drive from Southern California to Minnesota. At that time, it cost $25. For three mornings in a row —

from Flagstaff on — it was too cold for our car to start, and AAA promptly sent trucks to jump the battery and get us going. In less than a week, our $25 membership had saved us $75.

Sometimes we still leave the lights on or the car door ajar, and we'll come out to find the battery dead. Every year our AAA membership saves us in jump-starts several times the cost of dues.

AAA has a host of other services for motorists, as well — package tours, insurance, trip-planning service, member discounts and some of the best travel guides available. To join, look up the local AAA club in your phone book, or write AAA, 8111 Gatehouse Rd., Falls Church, VA 22047 ☎ 703/222-6334.

Other auto clubs offer benefits similar to AAA's. But before you join another, find out whether it offers road service as reliable as AAA's. And if you drive an RV, ask whether the emergency service covers RVs. Here are some of the clubs:

Amoco Motor Club — P.O. Box 9048, Des Moines, IA 50369 ☎ toll free 800/334-3300.

United States Auto Club — Motoring Division, P.O. Box 660460, Dallas, TX 75266 ☎ toll-free 800/348-2761.

Allstate Motor Club — P.O. Box 9025, Arlington Heights, IL 60006 ☎ toll-free 800/323-6282.

Chevron Travel Club — P.O. Box P, Concord, CA 94524 ☎ toll-free 800/222-0585.

Montgomery Ward Motor Club — 200 N. Martingale Rd., Schaumburg, IL 60173 ☎ toll-free 800/621-5151.

Exxon Travel Club — 4550 Dacoma, Rm. 865, Houston, TX 77092 ☎ 713/680-5723.

National Automobile Club — One Market Place, San Francisco, CA 94104 ☎ 415/777-4000. ·

Shell Motor Club — P.O. Box 60199, Chicago, IL 60660 ☎ toll-free 800/621-8663, in Illinois 312/338-7028.

GETTING SET FOR A TRIP

One of the things most auto clubs do for you is help plan the trip. Tell them where you want to go and what you want to see, and shortly they'll mail you a map of your whole trip with your route neatly outlined in colored pen. Some clubs also provide a written itinerary, with suggested stops or sights to see.

If you don't belong to an auto club, you have to do that planning for yourself. In any case, be sure you have planned the route very carefully and know where you're going. Get an atlas from your auto-insurance agent or a bookstore, or write tourism agencies in advance for maps of every state you plan to visit — their addresses follow Chapter 4, Armchair Travel. In addition to trip planning, here are some other things you need to do before you start:

• Make sure your car is in good mechanical shape, that the tires are properly filled and that you're starting off with a full tank of gas. It is very costly to have a breakdown or run out of gas on a freeway; and it is downright dangerous if you have to stop and change a tire.

• Make sure you have flares, a flashlight and tools you need to change a tire. If you're going somewhere in the winter, also carry chains and a shovel, candles, a tin can (for holding them and reflecting heat), matches, a blanket and snacks, like dried fruit or oatmeal cookies. A pair of leaf bags can serve as an emergency rain shelter or as an extra layer against the cold.

• Practice "combat packing." Make sure the things you need for an overnight in a motel are in a small bag on top of the luggage pile or at the front of the trunk. Things you don't need until you reach your destination — golf clubs, for example, or fancy clothes — should go in bags at the bottom. If your car is big enough, try not to stack bags over the spare tire or tool kit.

• Protect temperature-sensitive things like film, cosmetics or medicine. Don't keep them in the trunk. Instead, pack them in a carry-on bag you keep in the car.

• Carry extra car keys in a pants pocket or purse, or have your traveling companion carry them.

• Reserve a room ahead — at least for the first night. In summer, especially, the roads are crowded and "No Vacancy" signs start coming on in the middle of the afternoon.

• Get a good night's rest before you start.

Once you're on the road:

• Take a rest stop every two hours to avoid fatigue and muscle strain. Get out of the car, walk around, do some stretching exercises. If you're traveling with someone else who drives, trade off at the wheel.

• Top off your gas tank whenever you take a rest stop.

- Keep your seat straight up while you're driving to head off muscle fatigue, especially in the neck and shoulders. Keep your elbows close to your rib cage and your hands in 3 o'clock and 9 o'clock positions on the wheel.
- Eat light lunches. A heavy lunch will make you sleepy. Snack on fruit, and drink water. Don't change your normal caffeine intake — coffee or cola drinks.
- Talk to your passenger or play the radio to stay alert — preferably a talk show that keeps your mind busy.
- Open a window, even if you've got the air conditioning going. That will help get rid of cigarette smoke (which reduces the amount of oxygen in the car), or any fumes from your car's gas tank or fuel line. Use the outside-air setting rather than the recirculated air setting for the air conditioner.
- Make long drives in daylight. Poor light makes dusk statistically the most dangerous time to drive. At night, glare from oncoming traffic can blind you, and even if you've got good eyes, the stress level increases significantly.
- Don't push it. AAA says 400 or 500 miles of freeway driving, without stops for sightseeing, is all you should try in a day. If you're driving up mountains or on narrow backroads, don't try for more than 300 miles.

We like to get up early — 5 a.m. or thereabouts — get on the road before the traffic starts and stop for breakfast about an hour later. Then we'll drive, taking rest stops about every 100 miles, until mid-afternoon. We check in before the pool gets crowded, maybe take a short nap and then have a long, leisurely dinner. We find that way we've chewed up a lot of roadway without overstressing.

FREEWAYS AND OTHER WAYS

For those who enjoy driving vacations, the freeways are a fact of life.

Once, when we had nothing but time, we tried to drive from Minneapolis to San Francisco without ever getting on a freeway. We had a peaceful journey down the Minnesota River, tarried in the Black Hills, sped through Nevada's lonely basin-and-range country and wandered through the backroads of the Sacramento

Valley, up the backside of a mountain and into California's lovely wine country.

But once in Wyoming and again in California, we ran smack into mountains whose only passes carried Interstate 80. And in South Dakota, the maps told us that Interstate 90 was the only road exiting the state. We knew then that there is hardly anyplace you can go in America nowadays without getting onto a freeway.

Truly, the quickest way to get from City A to City B in the U.S. is on the freeways. But it can also be the quickest way to lose your mind, if you're not prepared for freeway driving. We don't believe freeway driving is as disorderly as its reputation indicates, but if you're not comfortable behind the wheel at speeds of 60-70 miles an hour, try to make your journeys on side roads. And there are lots of pleasurable side roads left.

Much of the old U.S. highway system is still in place, not upgraded to freeway standards. On many of those two-lane roadways, as well as on state routes almost everywhere, you can still go long distances, through America's small towns and rolling countryside, at a pace you'll find more comfortable.

Though you can be arrested for going too slow on a freeway, they are well-organized and usually predictable. Since there are no traffic lights, you can keep a steady pace for hours.

In most states there are comfortable roadside stops every 50 to 100 miles, with restrooms, picnic tables, maps, dog walks. Many are built at scenic or historic sites. Some have vending machines for pop and snacks. And before you pass a rest stop by, there is usually a sign telling you how far the next rest stop is.

Even states that have abolished billboards from their right-of-ways put up signs with pictures or glyphs, telling you what services are available at each exit, so you don't need to wonder whether you'll find things like gas, food or lodging when you turn off. There are turnoffs for scenic lookouts and historic markers.

If you're in trouble, there are usually milepost signs telling you where you are, and emergency roadside telephones every few miles. There are hospital and trauma center markers and weather signs. In California's Sierra, there are even signs telling truckers how to drive over the mountain ("Slight upgrade" — "let 'er drift" — "Downgrade ahead" — "Don't crowd it" and the like).

Truly, like your dog, the freeway can be your friend — though not a very interesting one.

CROSSING THE BORDER

Don't forget that when you cross the national border and plan to stay more than a few hours, you may have to prove your citizenship both ways — to the Mexican or Canadian authorities when you enter, and to U.S. authorities when you try to return. The best way to do that is with a passport, though they'll also accept such documents as birth or baptismal certificate, naturalization papers or Alien Registration Receipt Card.

Your home state driver's license is accepted for driving in both Canada and Mexico. Be sure to carry a vehicle registration form, as well. If you're driving a rented car, have a copy of the rental contract.

As proof of insurance in Canada, get a Canadian Non-Resident Insurance Card from your agent, or carry your insurance policy, itself. If you have a radar warning device — a fuzz-buster — leave it at home. Even if it's disconnected and in your trunk, Canadian police can confiscate them.

Otherwise, driving in Canada is mostly like driving in the United States.

DRIVING IN MEXICO

There's no need to worry about driving into Mexico, as long as you drive as carefully as you do at home and have the right papers.

Before you enter Mexico, ask your insurance agent whether your policy is any good there. Usually, you need to buy a Mexican insurance policy. If you're in a serious accident without Mexican insurance, the authorities can confiscate your car and jail you.

You can buy a Mexican insurance policy in advance from AAA offices in California, Arizona, New Mexico and Texas, or buy it at the border where you cross.

Except in Baja California, you'll also need a car permit to drive into Mexico. These are issued free at customs points; keep it with your insurance policy.

143

Roads in Mexico simply are not as good as those in the United States and Canada. Many are built without shoulders, and sometimes potholes are simply marked if there's been no money to repair them. Do not drive at night in Mexico — you could come across a black bull sleeping on the road, a boulder rolled onto the highway or a truck parked in your lane. You can understand why traffic seems to just creep along in some parts of Mexico.

On the other hand, drivers in crowded Mexico City go as fast as they can, just like their counterparts in Amsterdam, Paris and Rome — up to 60 mph. John Howells and Don Merwin, in their book, *Choose Mexico*, say, if you want to see Mexico City, park the car and take the Metro, buses or taxis. We think that's good advice for any large city, at home or abroad. Driving seems less hectic in smaller Mexican cities, however.

If you get in trouble driving Mexico's country roads, you can call on a "Green Angel." These are government trucks — painted green, obviously — that patrol every major route at least once a day. They carry gasoline and oil, spare parts and trained mechanics to help stranded motorists. You pay for the supplies, but the labor is free. In heavy tourist seasons, the army adds its own patrols. Look for Jeeps and other military vehicles along the roadway with signs: "Asistencia Turística".

DRIVING OVERSEAS

In Scandinavian countries, you are required to drive with your headlights on, even in the daytime.

If you're entering a traffic circle in England, you have to give way to cars already in the circle. But in France, the car entering the circle has the right-of-way.

In Great Britain, drivers are expected to make way for sheep and cattle in the roadways. In the Alps, you are supposed to sound your horn frequently when approaching a curve.

And don't think that driving on the left side, as you must do in Great Britain and a number of other places — including one U.S. possession — will be a breeze. Once we got a car in Jamaica, and every time we tried to turn on the lights, the windshield got washed. We tried to shift gears, and only managed to bang our knuckles against the right window. After an evening of jack-rabbit driving through the streets of Ocho Ríos with clean windows but without lights, we turned the car in.

Remember that the auto's controls, as well as the roads, are turned around. If you've been used to shifting gears with your right hand all your life, it takes some practice to drive the opposite way. We advise getting an automatic shift.

Truly, driving overseas can be breathtaking — especially in major cities, where every driver seems to close his eyes and push down hard on the horn and the gas pedal.

We would never recommend having a car in cities like Rome, Paris or Amsterdam. On the other hand, driving through the countryside puts you closer to the people than you can get any other way. It's not practical to take your own car abroad, unless you're staying permanently. So you'll no doubt have to rent a car. We have friends who follow this policy: The first time, take a tour; after that, rent a car.

In most places, your home-state driver's license will get you by overseas. But at least three countries — Japan, Spain and South Korea — require you to have an international driver's license. And many others require you to carry a translation of your license, which you have to get at the local U.S. embassy.

Whether you're a member or not, $5 will buy you an international driver's license — which is printed in nine languages — from most local AAA offices. You need a valid state license and a passport photo. Since you have to appear in person, you cannot get one by mail.

Just as in Mexico, your regular auto-insurance policy doesn't meet the requirements of many other countries. You can buy short-term policies where you rent your car, or get one at most AAA offices that covers liability and property damage, collision and comprehensive. If you are an AAA member driving overseas, you'll find free road service, towing and other important AAA services available to you from foreign auto clubs that offer reciprocity. For a list of foreign clubs and the services they provide, ask AAA for the booklet *Offices to Serve You Abroad*.

In some countries, because of insurance restrictions, auto-rental agencies won't rent to anyone over 60. Other countries have legal maximum ages for driving. In the Philippines, for example, it's 65.

To avoid disappointment, ask your travel agent before you go to get all the forms you'll need, to check out all the driving restrictions and get you a printed set of local driving laws and customs.

RENTING A CAR

One place where the AARP card does not get you much is at car-rental agencies.

We recently phoned Avis to check on renting a car in New York. The price for that week, we were told, was $175. Then we called back on AARP's special toll-free number. The AARP rate for that week, the lady said, was $176. That same kind of car at Thrifty, without any discounts at all, was $160. It started us thinking.

We tried it again for London. Avis's international desk quoted a regular rate of £129; AAA members got a rate of £116, a 10 percent discount. Avis's AARP desk, however, quoted a rate of £276. Thrifty's rate was £62.

In Chicago, AARP members rated only a little higher among several car- rental firms. The explanation is fairly easy:

The three big auto-rental companies that have separate AARP desks and that AARP touts in its membership material, quote their senior-citizen discounts off regular, full prices. But almost every week, the companies have specials going for the general public.

That means members who use the special AARP toll-free numbers for Avis, Hertz and National are not told about these deep-discount specials unless they ask. These desks do not quote members the lowest rate available.

Misleading advertising and false rates quoted by auto-rental companies are becoming a national scandal — even their executives admit that. What is even more misleading is AARP's promise of whopping discounts on auto rentals — up to 25 percent — from Avis, Hertz and National. The truth is that discounts offered to AARP members by Dollar and Thrifty are better than AARP's favored three. Avis and Hertz give even better discounts to AAA members than they do to those of AARP.

A senior would be foolish to rent a car from Avis, which quotes higher rates for AARP members at some locations than for the general public, a survey by *The Mature Traveler* newsletter indicated.

And in our spot-checks of London and New York (JFK) rental rates, and another of Chicago, unheralded Thrifty consistently came out the lowest, whatever your age.

The message is clear: if you need to rent a car, whether in the U.S. or overseas, get on the phone and shop the toll-free 800 numbers — or make sure your travel agent has done so. Numbers for the major rental companies are below.

WHAT TO SHOP FOR

Auto-rental companies will not lie to you — they just won't tell you everything unless you ask.

For rentals in the United States and Canada, for example, they'll quote a rate that doesn't include any tax or extras. Extras can be insurance that you may or not need (check with your insurance agent), gas charges or drop-off charges. In short, what you are quoted will probably not be the "drive-out" rate.

In England, one of the things they don't mention, for example, is that there's a 15 percent tax on top of everything. The tax on a rented car in Spain is 33 1/3 percent.

So you'll hear things like, "Your weekly rate is £87, less your 10 percent discount." You're never told that to drive out with the car, it will cost you close to £91, even with that discount. Before you make the reservation for overseas rental, insist that the clerk tells you the drive-out rate — including any extras.

Extras can include:

• Fuel service fee — If you take it out with a full tank, they want it back with a full tank, or otherwise they'll charge an exorbitant price for the gas.

• Drop charge — Unless you return the car to the same place you rented it, they'll charge you extra to fetch it back.

• Insurance — If you are in an accident or your rental car is stolen, the Collision Damage Waiver (CDW) lets you walk away without extra cost. Without the coverage, the rental company can charge your credit card up to the full value of the car. Check with your insurance agent to see whether your own policy will cover, instead — about 60 percent of auto insurance policies do, as well as some credit cards. Other coverages the rental car company may try to sell you that you may not need are Personal Accident Insurance (which takes care of medical bills) and Personal Effects Options (that covers things stolen from your car). Turn them all down if you have other insurance.

Insist that you're quoted a price in terms of the local currency. Auto-rental companies we talked to used exchange rates for London that varied from $1.60 to $1.87 to the pound — the lower the exchange rate, the better their rates sound. But local currency — not U.S. dollars — is the only common denominator in the auto rental business.

When you're shopping, the reservation clerk will ask you for the exact date, even the time, you want to pick up the car. If your plans aren't firm, pull a date out of the hat — and make it the same date for all the other companies you call.

Always ask about a comparable kind of car, and remember that the rental companies each use different terms — subcompacts, economies, standards, mid-sizes, full sizes, luxury, whatever. If you want a Cadillac, specify a Cadillac; if the company has only Lincolns, that's okay.

When we shop, we specify "the littlest car you've got." That's varied from a Ford Fiesta up to an Olds Cutlass — both at a subcompact price.

Rental rates, even for the same car rented by the same company, will vary widely week by week, location by location and season by season. But get a general idea from your shopping of the company that offers the lowest rate for the season and the place you want to go.

Then begin asking about discounts.

AUTO-RENTAL DEALS FOR SENIORS

Always ask for the discounts. Nobody pays full rate in this highly competitive market. Auto-rental companies that don't offer you some kind of discount don't want your business very much.

Almost all the major auto-rental companies offer discounts for AARP members, as well as those of AAA, American Legion, AOPA, VFW and a host of other organizations. A few, like Budget Car & Truck Rental, also offer discounts to members of Mature Outlook, September Days and other seniors' organizations.

Some airline clubs for seniors (see Chapter 15, Flying) also have tie-ins with car-rental companies. None that we could find, however, offers discounts to seniors who don't belong to anything.

Here are some of the major auto-rental companies that give senior discounts:

• Alamo — Every location gives an AARP discount, but the percentage varies from city to city. In Chicago, for example, it ranged from 20 percent off (weekly) to 38 percent off (daily). No overseas locations. ☎ 800/327-9633.

• Avis — Gives AARP discounts in some cities, though local specials for the general public are often priced lower. (See the tables at the end of this chapter). ☎ 800/331-1212 (U.S.), ☎ 800/331-2112 (international), 800/331-1800 (AARP).

• Budget — AARP and Mature Outlook discounts vary by location. No overseas rental discounts, though regular rates were among the lowest quoted. ☎ 800/527-0700.

• Dollar — A 10 percent across-the-board AARP discount. No discounts overseas. ☎ 800/421-6868.

• Hertz — Offers varying AARP discounts at all locations, including overseas. ☎ 800/654-3131, 800/654-3001 (international), 800/654-2200 (AARP).

• National — Offers 10-to-20 percent AARP discounts in most locations. ☎ 800/227-7368 (U.S.), 800/227-3876 (international), 800/227-7368 (AARP).

• Thrifty — Has an AARP rate that varies by locations, including the lowest overseas rates we were quoted. ☎ 800/367-2277.

IN SUMMARY:

— An auto-club membership saves many times the cost of dues.
— If you're not comfortable driving at 60-70 mph, stay off the freeways.
— Check your auto insurance coverage before crossing the border.
— Ask your travel agent for help if you're renting a car overseas.
— Use toll-free 800 numbers to price-shop before you reserve a rental car.
— Always ask for the discounts.

Travel Tool
★ ★ ★

SOME COMPARATIVE RATES FOR RENTAL CARS

In a recent survey, *The Mature Traveler* newsletter phoned car rental companies' toll-free 800 numbers and was quoted these rates for subcompact rental cars in three locations. The domestic rates do not include taxes, which rental companies will not quote. The London rates, stated in pounds, include a 15 percent tax and are probably "drive-out" rates. Rates vary weekly and by season, and should be regarded only as an indication of which companies offer mature travelers the best deals. Note that some companies' regular rates are lower than others' AARP rates.

	Daily		Weekly	
	Reg.	AARP	Reg.	AARP
IN CHICAGO (O'HARE):				
Alamo	$40	$25	$124	$100
Avis	57	35	125	119
Budget	53	43	115	115
Dollar	40	36	180	162
Hertz	65	41	149	134
National	57	51	158	142
Thrifty	32	30	180	160
IN NEW YORK (JFK):				
Alamo (no location)				
Avis	$43	$45	$175	$176
Budget	53	46	179	179
Dollar	53	48	189	170
Hertz	58	45	195	175
National	54	49	384	288
Thrifty	44	33	160	160
IN LONDON (GATWICK)*:				
Avis	£53	£53	£129	£156
Budget	21**	21**	106	106
Dollar	30	30	121	121
Hertz	23**	18**	121	121
National	21**	17**	101	91
Thrifty	8	8	62	62

*In pounds sterling.
**Plus mileage charge.

★ ★ ★
Travel Tool
★ ★ ★

INTERNATIONAL ROAD SIGNS

Most countries use a standard international sign system, which is a series of pictures that almost speak for themselves. Here are the most important ones:

Danger warnings/

Left curve

Right curve

Zigzag or switchback, starting to the left

Zigzag or switchback, starting to the right

Steep descent (1 in 10)

Dip

Slippery road

Loose gravel

Falling rocks

Pedestrian crossing

Road narrows

Road narrows at left

Draw bridge

Road leads to quay or river

Uneven road

Signs giving restrictions/

No entry

Closed to vehicles in both directions

Closed to all motor vehicles except cycles

No motorcycles

No cycles

No pedestrians

No handcarts

No delivery trucks

No vehicles with trailers except semi-trailers or single-axle trailers

Quantity of inflammable substances restricted

Stopping and parking signs/

No parking

No stopping
or parking

Limited-duration
parking

Parking

Limited-duration
parking

Signs that must be obeyed/

Turn left only

Straight ahead
only

Turn right only

Turn right or
straight ahead only

Pass this side

Compulsory
bike lane

Compulsory
foot path

Compulsory
bridleway

Compulsory
minimum speed

End of
compulsory
minimum speed

Signs before intersections/

Traffic circle

Junction with
minor roads

Junction with
minor road

Junction with
minor road

Junction with
minor road

Signs at railroad crossings/

Railroad crossing
with gates or
barricades

Railroad crossing
without barriers

Intersection with
streetcar line

One-track
crossing without
gates

Multi-track
crossing
without gates

CHAPTER 11

THE RV LIFESTYLE

| It's As Much a Lifestyle as a Means of Getting There |

For the retiree, with almost limitless time to roam, RVing can be as much a lifestyle as a means of travel. RV campers are modern-day Gypsies, moving from place to place, sometimes in groups, sometimes as singles, seemingly as the mood takes them.

"RV," of course, means "recreation vehicle" — motorhomes, travel trailers, truck campers, fifth-wheels, van campers and the like — those mostly self-contained campers with galleys, beds, toilets, TVs and whatever else you require to make life comfortable on the road.

RVers will drive 300 miles on the spur of the moment to take part in a rally. And they will just as casually plan a 3,000-mile swing up the coast from Los Angeles to Seattle, then back through Las Vegas, or take an eight-week tour of the United States. If they want to stay awhile with old friends, they'll take a ninth week, or if they're bored, they'll come home early.

They'll drive fearlessly into untracked desert or deep into Mexico. They'll even fly overseas to RV across Europe or Australia. And wherever they go, they'll go visiting. There's nothing RVers love more than sitting around a campfire visiting with one another.

WHY SENIORS GO RVING

A vast majority of all RVers in America are 49ers-plus — 72 percent of all RV trips are taken by seniors, according to AARP.

And RVing rates No. 1 as seniors' favorite way to travel — 18 percent of all trips taken by seniors are in RVs.

RVing makes it possible to visit your friends and relatives around the country without really imposing on them too much — you can live in your rig instead of their bedroom.

And RVing is probably the least expensive way to see America — the cost of an RV trip is one-quarter to one-half that of a comparable vacation by other means. The reasons are simple: you pay $10-$20 for a campsite compared to motel bills of $30-$40 a night. You fix many of your own meals instead of having to eat out. And if you haul in beside a wilderness stream and fish for your dinner, there's no cost at all.

RVing is not necessarily just a wilderness adventure, either. Almost everywhere in America there are modern RV campgrounds with things like laundries, hot showers, posh lounges, swimming pools, miniature golf, free movies, tours and activities schedules that almost match a cruiseship's. Classy RV resorts offer tennis, horseback riding and great restaurants. Indeed, the manager of a huge South Texas campground, where RV snowbirds from the North nest for several months in the winter, told us, "We run this place like a cruiseship — something going on all the time."

There are an estimated 11,000 RV campgrounds in the United States and Canada, in the cities as well as in the country — next door to Opryland in Nashville, across from Disneyland in Anaheim, Calif., just a short drive from Epcot Center, Sea World, Disney World and the other attractions in the Orlando, Fla., area. Anywhere you want to go, there's a modern RV campground where you can pull in, plug in and be off to see the sights.

The appeal of traveling in an RV, especially for retired people, is its freedom. In an RV, you are always at home and on your own schedule. There's no need to pack or unpack. You carry your hotel room on your back. Your kitchen is always open and serving special meals. You'll have a shower — maybe even a bathtub — your own water supply, heating, air-conditioning. You'll be able to live self-contained in all but the smallest RVs for weeks on the road.

But why would you want to, when you can stop at a modern campground, park your rig at a tree-shaded campsite, plug in your electricity, water intake and sewage outlet and go take a dip in the pool or a hot shower?

Many retirees become "snowbirds" — following the sun in their RVs to Florida, Arizona or Texas for the winter, then returning north in the summer. Some are even full-timers — living all year in their RVs. Most, though, keep permanent homes somewhere, and travel perhaps half the time seeing their country.

RVers are also a friendlier lot than most — there's a camaraderie that develops around a campfire, a shared pot of coffee and a shared hobby that's not associated with many other kinds of travel. Through their clubs, caravans and camporees, RVers tend to keep in touch with each other no matter how far apart they live. For that reason, RVing appeals to many singles — mostly widowed or divorced. They find it impossible to be lonely in the company of other RVers.

On the downside, if you're a loner or have trouble meeting strangers, you may not like RVing — a large part of the fun in staying at a campground is making friends with fellow campers.

RVing is also not for you if your travel time is limited or if you want to get somewhere in a hurry. RVs are bigger than autos, usually traveling in the slow lanes. There's a lot of temptation to dawdle along the way, and along popular routes you usually have to pull in early to make sure you get a campsite. Retirees will have that kind of time — many others don't.

The initial cost of RVing is pretty heavy, too, especially for mature travelers who may not want to rough it too much. Though you can get into a basic tent-trailer for just a few thousand dollars, a comfortable big rig easily runs up to $50,000 (some over $100,000), and even a smaller used RV that's reasonably livable can cost $12,000 to $15,000.

As we said, RVing is as much a lifestyle as a way to travel. And whether that lifestyle suits you is something you can debate around the campfire, with marshmallows and a hot cup of coffee, into the early hours.

You'll never be sure until you try it.

TRYING IT ONCE

If you've never traveled in an RV and think you might want to, the best way to get started is with friends. Most RVs sleep four to six people, and for just a weekend, there's plenty of room.

With friends, you can get pointers on driving an RV (which is wider and higher than the auto you may be used to), you'll hear their views on the merits of different kinds of RVs, and you'll learn some campground protocol right off the bat.

If you don't know anyone who owns an RV, rent one for a trial weekend. There are RV rental centers near every large city. If one isn't listed in your phone book, send $4.75 for the booklet *Who's Who in RV Rentals*, published by the Recreation Vehicle Rental Association, 3251 Old Lee Hwy., Ste. 500, Fairfax, VA 22030. The directory lists more than 250 RV rental centers in the U.S. and Canada, along with rates, deposit information and size of RVs available.

For a trial run, we suggest you get a mini-motorhome. If you can handle an automobile, you probably can handle a 19- to 21-foot RV like a Winnebago LeSharo or a small Coachman. Don't rent any kind of trailer model the first time — though there are some real advantages to having an RV you can unhitch, you have to get your truck or auto rigged with a trailer hitch, and you'll need some practice driving with it. The rental fee for a small RV will run $200 or more for a weekend. You'll also have to stock the RV with groceries, bedding and utensils.

Ask the rental agent endless questions about how to handle the rig, how to fill the water tank, how to dump the sewage, how to handle the propane tank and so on. Also ask him about good campgrounds to go within a few hours' drive.

Don't head for a wilderness camp the first time. Instead, find a commercial campground like a Kampground of America (KOA), where camping will be easier and help will be close if you need it. Pick a place 200 miles or less from your home — you don't want to spend the whole weekend driving or arrived too tired to enjoy the experience.

When you get to the campground, just park, walk in and register, as you would at a motel. On that first trip, ask for "full hookups" — those are electric, water and sewer connections.

Even if you don't need them for a short weekend, you'll learn how they operate for your longer trips.

At the registration desk, you'll be assigned a campsite and told how to drive to it. Most campsites include a picnic table and a fire ring or barbecue so you can take your meals outdoors. There's likely to be a convenience store on the campground, where you can buy supplies you forgot to pack.

On some campgrounds there are movies every night in the rec hall, bingo and other games and campfire programs. Some campers get their "campfire fix" simply by visiting other campers' fire ring and having a cup of coffee.

It's a good idea, especially in the summer, to call ahead for reservations, just as you would for a motel. To find a good campground, borrow a campground directory from the rental agent, or get one of your own. You can get a free *KOA Directory, Road Atlas and Camping Guide* — one of the most complete — from any KOA campground you pass, and they can also make reservations for you at any other KOA down the road. AAA *CampBook* directories are also free if you're an AAA member.

Other good directories you can buy at bookstores are Woodall's *Campground Directory of North America* and Rand McNally's *Campground Guide*.

Choose a fairly large campground if you can — one with 200 spaces or more — for a look at typical campground life. The larger the campground, the more people you're likely to meet and the more you're likely to learn. If you're having a problem with your rented rig, ask the campground manager how to fix it. Find out about campground activities, and meet some other campers. Don't be bashful — walk around and talk to others. Tell them you're new to RVing — RVers like nothing better than to fill a tenderfoot with the joys of their chosen hobby.

When you see an RV you like, knock on the door and ask to see inside. Ask the owners what it's like to live in that kind of rig, and whether they'd buy that model again. If you see a piece of equipment you like — a special stove, a fold-up picnic table, whatever — ask about that, too.

Around the campfire or in the rec hall, listen to the stories RVers swap about where they've been and the kind of RV activities available.

It shouldn't take more than that first weekend to know whether you'll like the RV lifestyle, what kind of rig you want to buy and what you want to do in it.

If RVing is for you, start shopping for your own rig, and begin reading an RV magazine regularly — a good one you can pick up on magazine racks is *Trailer Life* ($18/year, P.O. Box 55793, Boulder, CO 80322-5793). Two good guides that will tell you about the kinds of RVs available, floor plans, sizes and approximate costs are *Trailer Life's RV Buyer's Guide* ($4.95, TL Enterprises, Inc., 29901 Agoura Rd., Agoura, CA 91301) and *Woodall's RV Buyer's Guide* ($6.70, Woodall Publishing Co., 100 Corporate, N. Suite 100, Bannock Burn, IL 60015-1255).

Attend RV shows; there you can compare all different kinds of RVs parked side by side, and talk to the experts. Watch your newspaper for show dates in your town, or write RVIA, P.O. Box 2999, Reston, VA 22090, for a current listing of shows around the country.

WHAT CAMPERS DO

Anything you can do in an auto, you can also do in your RV — and then some.

Whoever heard of an auto caravan, or an auto camporee, or boondocking in the family car?

Those are some of the things RVers do.

True, some people travel in their RVs as they would in the family auto — touring or base-camping — and using campgrounds as others would use motels. Touring is simply driving from point to point in your RV — perhaps visiting Sister Kate in San Francisco from your home in Illinois — and overnighting at campgrounds. Base-camping is heading for a destination campground — say, one at Yellowstone Park or Kissimmee, Fla., near Orlando — and spending the week daytripping around the area. You can take that kind of vacation in an auto, too.

Here are some things RVers do that make their kind of camping very special:

Rallying — A popular weekend pastime for RVers is road rallying; drivers of those big rigs mull their clues and time their checkpoints just as if they were driving swift Porsches or feisty little Alfas. Rallies are organized by both RV clubs and individual campgrounds. Often a rally is planned as part of a weekend camporee.

Caravaning — Caravaning is how club members travel as a group. RVers get together by the 20s and 30s, even the 50s, and drive nose-to-tail to the destination they've selected. Caravaning is a popular way to tour Mexico — there's lots of safety in numbers, they feel. But caravaning goes on everywhere, even overseas. Weekend caravans are common, and some RV groups plan caravans lasting up to several weeks. Caravaners usually get special rates at campgrounds.

Camporees — Camporees are simply jamborees organized for RVers. They can last for days or weeks. A group organizing a camporee reserves the campground and plans the activities — which usually include dancing, sightseeing and other entertainment. Smaller camporees can be on a campground; many are on public sites that hold more vehicles, like state fair grounds.

Boondocking — You just find a place in the open — maybe up a canyon or beside a nice stream — and park. There aren't any hookups — after all, your RV has holding tanks for sewage and water that will last awhile. And there isn't any cost. Many RVers boondock in one spot all winter, going into town only to replenish supplies and dump their sewage. Some install solar panels on their rigs so boondocking won't drain their batteries. The fun in boondocking is when several thousand RVers do it together — as in Quartzite, Slab City or Laughlin — and the desert becomes one giant campground.

Snowbirding — One special joy in RVing is that you can pick your seasons, beating the heat of summer by moving into Canada or the North Woods, fleeing the winter blizzards into Arizona, Texas or Florida. People who do that are called "Snowbirds" (except in south Texas, where they're called "Winter Texans" and become part of community life).

You've almost got to be an RV insider to know when some of these things are going on — you can drive a long way in the desert heat to Quartzite in December and find absolutely nothing there. Lots of activities are organized by word-of-mouth around the campfires.

The best way to get in on this RV grapevine is to join something.

WHAT CAMPERS JOIN

As much as they like their independence, RVers are notorious joiners. The clubs they belong to multiply the fun.

When you see a line of 20 or 30 of those silver-canister Airstreams moving down the highway, you're watching the Wally Byam Caravan Club International in action. It's the oldest and best-known of the RV clubs, originally founded by Airstream Corp. to sell travel trailers by promoting RVing. Today, almost every RV manufacturer sponsors a club that gives members reasons to gather (camporees, rallies and the like), trade notes and have fun. But don't contact them — they'll contact you, the instant you buy an RV.

In recent years, the manufacturers' clubs have been upstaged in both numbers and variety of activities by The Good Sam (for "good Samaritan") Club. Good Sam is easily the biggest club for RVers, with close to a million members. And why not join if you own an RV? At a minimum, your $15 yearly dues gets you a 10 percent discount at 1,600 Good Sam-approved campgrounds around the country, plus a free magazine, *Hiway Herald*.

Good Sam organizes all kinds of national and regional activities for members — called "Samborees" — reasons for RVers to gather and have a party. Good Sam runs a trip-routing service, a mail-forwarding service, a telephone service, a lost-key service, a lost-pet service, an emergency road service, a credit-card protection plan and more. And it offers member discounts on everything from film developing to magazines to RV repair.

And there are member discounts on tours — including cruises and overseas trips ("Caraventures" and "Good Sam-tours").

If you get the idea Good Sammers are supposed to have fun RVing, you're right. And Good Sam is the best way we know to plug in on the RVers' grapevine.

For membership information, write The Good Sam Club at P.O. Box 500, Agoura, CA 91301, or ☎phone toll-free 800/423-5061.

Most other clubs are operated by RVers who are on the road a lot, and they don't even have telephone numbers. But they all have little bulletins that promote their events, carry gossipy news about members, run travel-partner ads and help you keep in touch with RV buddies. Here's how to contact some of the other major clubs:

Loners on Wheels (LOW) — For RVers who are single — widowed, divorced, whatever — and just can't stay off the road. The club's 3,000 members camp together, rally together, caravan together. About the only thing they don't do together is share the same RV — LOW is not a matchmaking service, and members who pair up have to leave the club. Many LOWs are full-timers. There's a chatty newsletter in which members keep in touch with each other and share their activities. Write Dick March, Loners on Wheels, 808 Lester St., Poplar Bluff, MO 63901.

Loners of America (LOA) — A new group, with about 1,200 members in 28 chapters, that split off from Loners on Wheels. It's program is similar to LOW's, and there is a lively newsletter. Like LOW, LOA has strict rules about maintaining a single status. In summers, write Lorraine Shannon, Office Manager, Loners of America, Inc., Rte. 2, Box 85D, Ellsinore, MO 63937. In winters, write her at 191 Villa Del Rio Blvd., Boca Raton, FL 33432.

Friendly Roamers — This is what the Loners join after they marry or otherwise pair up and are no longer eligible for LOW or LOA membership, but want to keep RVing. For a newsletter and infomation send a stamped (45 cents) self-addressed envelope to Dot Sanford, P.O. Box 3393, North Shore, CA 92254-0968.

Escapees — With more than 12,000 members, mostly full-time RVers, this club sponsors a series of 11 co-op campgrounds stretching from Washington State to Florida. The campgrounds are member-owned, and members camp free or rent lots from each other at extremely low rates — $3 to $6 in most cases — as they travel. Mostly, these serve as social centers where full-timers gather. Write Kay and Joe Peterson, Escapees Club, Rte. 5, Box 310, Livingston, TX 77351 ☎ 409/327-8873.

Family Motorcoach Association — A club for those with self-contained, self-propelled motorhomes. A major club activity is promoting RV rallies and camporees around the country. Write P.O. Box 44144, Cincinnati, OH 45244.

Handicap Travel Club — Promotes RV travel for those with physical handicaps. Write Jean Kincaid, Rte. 1, Box 77, Lewis, KS 67552.

WHERE CAMPERS GO

RVers, of course, go everywhere that roads are built. But there are some special places where you'll find them as thick as bees on a hive. Twenty thousand RVs parked together in the desert at Quartzite, Ariz., is an awesome sight. Or is it 30,000?

"I couldn't count — 20,000 or 30,000 campers," one fellow who ran a concession there told us. "Looks all the same to me."

If there's a yellow brick road for RVers, surely it is U.S. 95 south from Las Vegas, Nev., to Yuma, Ariz. Along that road and its alternate, Arizona S.R. 95, places like Bullhead City, Lake Havasu, Quartzite and Blythe are legendary for sun-worshiping snowbirds. In one direction is the snowbird capital of Slab City, in another are Phoenix, Tucson and the Sun Cities, largest retirement communities in the United States.

In Texas, around McAllen, Harlingen and Brownsville, 100,000 or more "Winter Texans" — almost all RVers — more than double the population of the Lower Rio Grande Valley. And from there they regularly caravan into Mexico.

And in Florida and the Gulf Coast, RVing snowbirds spread throughout the land, though they don't cluster by the tens of thousands as they do in the West. Here are some of RVers favorite spots:

Bullhead City, Ariz. — The RV gambling capital of the country. It's right across the Colorado River from Laughlin, Nev., about 100 miles south of Las Vegas. Laughlin is for low-rollers: no big showroom stars, just high-paying slots, low-cost Bingo and Keno games and dollar blackjack tables. There's little in Laughlin but hotel-casinos; cheaper lodging, restaurants and campgrounds are on the Bullhead side. RV snowbirds are flocking to Bullhead in increasing numbers, and making Laughlin the fastest growing city in Nevada — with a gambling volume smaller only than Las Vegas's and Reno's. Most RVers camp in Bullhead and cross to the casinos in darting little shuttle boats that always seem to be waiting. If you want to camp on the Nevada side, the casinos let boondocking RVers use their parking lots free as long as their water supply and their money holds out.

That could be all winter, because nobody there forces you to play, the meals are cheap and the drinking is often free.

Quartzite, Ariz. — Just a dusty, dry place on the desert where U.S. 95 crosses Interstate 10, about 80 miles north of Yuma. It's a little town of about 500 souls, until January, when up to 30,000 RVers converge on the place and spread out on the desert as far as the eye can see. Rockhounders started it, gathering there for a few days to trade stones and stories. Over the years the "Main Event," as RVers call it, just grew and grew until it's become perhaps the largest — and certainly the craziest — flea market in America. You can buy virtually anything that will fit inside your RV at Quartzite, all created or at least sold by your fellow RVers.

Quartzite is the closest thing there is to a national RV convention. All the clubs have hospitality tents at Quartzite, and lately RV vendors have been setting up booths there — RV makers and outfits like Coleman, KOA and even individual campgrounds come to Quartzite to sell their wares.

Though many RVers camp at Quartzite all winter, the two-week Main Event occurs suddenly at the end of January and early in February every year. It's virtually unannounced — we've never seen a written notice that it's about to take place. There's no real organization, no public relations department to send out notices, no host committee to assign credentials — Quartzite just happens. RVers simply know when to be there.

Florida — Five million RVers visit Florida every year and the Orlando area in central Florida is a magnet, with at least 33 RV parks and campgrounds. With a moderate climate all year, Orlando has a 12-month season, as well as attractions like Epcot Center, Disney World and Sea World to draw visitors. One of the most lavish RV resorts in the Orlando area is Fort Wilderness, with 1,200 campsites near Epcot in Lake Buena Vista. In addition to the lure of nearby attractions, Fort Wilderness offers fishing, sailboating, horseback riding and walking trails across its 750-acre spread. You can drive your own rig there, or rent one of 400 RVs that are parked their permanently. Write Fort Wilderness Resort, P.O. Box 10040, Lake Buena Vista, FL 32830, or call ☎ 407/934-7639.

Slab City — Where on earth is Slab City? You might as well ask where on earth is Niland — it's no harder to find one than the other, though Slab City was once featured on CBS's *60 Minutes*.

To find Niland, you look on a California map in the direction of the Salton Sea. And to find Slab City, you go to Niland and follow the RVs a few miles east. There you'll find what's left of the base Gen. George Patton used during World War II to train his tank divisions. Now it's just a decaying network of roads and slabs where barracks used to sit. But boondockers think it's RV paradise — a few thousand of them winter-in there every year, and a growing number come and go. Just find the place and haul your rig onto an empty slab. It's absolutely free.

Why do RVers congregate there? John Howells, for his book *Retirement Choices*, asked a Slab City winter resident, who replied, "We feel safer here by far than in the city. Here, we all watch out for each other. If a troublemaker tries to move in, he either changes his attitude or leaves because of isolation. No one steals or vandalizes, even though we might leave our rigs here for a week or two while we go visiting elsewhere."

Can you say that about camping in Central Park?

CAMPING OVERSEAS

Travelers from North America can fly overseas, pick up a rental RV and see the countryside at their leisure and at considerably less expense than if they were staying in hotels. There are an increasing number of tour packages like this, both for groups that will caravan together and for those who'll travel alone.

The most popular starting place for a European camping trip is London. You drive for a day through the Kentish countryside to the Dover coast, getting used to your new rig, then take a ferry across the channel to wherever you're going in Europe.

Now tour packages are available for New Zealand, China and Australia RV trips, as well.

RVing overseas, especially in Europe, is a different kind of camping experience than it is in America. For one thing, European camping vehicles are smaller than Americans', because gas is more expensive. And those who've camped in Europe say the campgrounds aren't as up-to-date as those in America. A Britisher touring the West with an RV group told us most European campgrounds have no showers, no hookups and no sanitary dump sites.

164

"There's nothing like KOA in Europe," he said. "You carry the loo around with you in an aluminum tube."

On the other hand, because European RVs are smaller, you can get onto the back roads and through narrow mountain passes to scenic places most tourists never get to visit. To find out about those places off the beaten path, of course, you'll need a good insider guidebook or a tour caravan with a knowledeable guide or wagonmaster.

Many of the clubs mentioned above organize RV trips abroad for their members — Good Sam has a constant series of tours and trips, as does AARP.

If you don't belong to a club, Kampgrounds of America (KOA) has a year-round calendar of escorted RV caravan trips to Great Britain, Europe, Australia and New Zealand, as well as Alaska, the U.S. mainland and Mexico. KOA also arranges unescorted individual RV tours through these countries.

A month's caravaning in Scandinavia, for example, costs $4,749 a couple, not including airfare, gasoline or groceries — you'd make it on less than $100 a day apiece, a real value for an overseas tour. An additional person sharing the same rig would cost only $1,179. Other European destinations for KOA caravaning tours include Greece and Turkey, the Iberian Peninsula, the Soviet Union and several other countries.

Write KOA Tours, P.O. Box 30558, Billings, MT 59114, or ☎ phone toll-free 800/225-5562.

Another, less-expensive way to travel abroad in an RV is through a program called International Camper Exchange (ICE), run by a retired surgeon and his wife in North Bend, Wash. Bill and Betty Topping arrange RV swaps between Americans and Europeans. Toppings tell us you will save up to $2,000 on a two-week exchange, and get to see Europe at your own pace, to boot.

Toppings start setting up the complicated swaps a year in advance. To start the process, you become an ICE member at $60 a year. You'll fill out a form describing your rig, your preferred travel dates and where you want to go. ICE compiles applicants from here and applicants from there into blocks of 20, and then mails out the listings. Then you write a compatible family abroad to firm up the swap.

"The concept of swapping is not new," Toppings tell us. "ICE is a result of our travels through swap-exchanges in continental Europe and England . . . We find that our retirement income will only permit going our way — camping. Swapping is the only way we know to do that."

They have plans to expand the ICE program to New Zealand and Australia.

For information send a stamped, self-addressed #10 envelope to International Camper Exchange, Inc., at P.O. Box 947, North Bend, WA 98045, or call ☎ 206/888-9382.

RV DEALS FOR 49ERS-PLUS

Relatively few campgrounds offer special discounts for 49ers-plus — after all, most RV campers are seniors, which makes the regular rates senior rates. Even so, we come across a few campgrounds from time to time that have small discounts for seniors.

One such is Burnaby Cariboo RV Park on the northeast edge of Vancouver, which gives a 10 percent discount to campers 60 and older. There's also a special weekly rate for reverse snowbirds — those fleeing the summer heat of the South and Southwest. And as a bonus, Burnaby Cariboo will store your RV for only $5 (CDN) a day if you want to hop the cruiseships to Alaska, most of which leave from Vancouver. For a brochure, write Burnaby Cariboo RV Park, 8765 Cariboo Pl., Burnaby, BC V3N 4T2, or call ☎ 604/420-1722.

You're likely to find some senior discounts also at campgrounds along the snowbird routes — Interstate 95 into Florida, I-35 to Texas and I-15, I-25 and I-40 to the Southwest. These are campgrounds trying to get you to stop there for a week or two coming and going. Here are some other good deals for RVers:

KOA Value Card — Though it's for any RVer, a good deal is the KOA Value Card, which gives you 10 percent off regular rates at any of 650 KOA Kampgrounds. Many of the 1,600 Good Sam campgrounds also give 10 percent discounts when you show a KOA Value Card. You pay $6 for the card at any KOA you stop at, and the discount applies immediately. Or send your $6 to Kampgrounds of America, P.O. Box 30558, Billings, MT 59114.

By the way, though their corporate office discourages it, many KOAs also accept Good Sam cards. The point is that the RV insider always carries one card or the other, and never pays more than 90 percent of the rack rate at a campground.

Golden Age passes to parks — Travelers 62 or older who carry Golden Age passes get free admission to national parks and wildlife refuges, plus 50 percent discounts on park user fees, like overnight RV camping. Golden Age passes are accepted as proof of age for discounts or free camping at most state-park campgrounds, as well. You have to apply in person for a pass and prove your age — an AARP card won't do. Go to any office of the National Park Service, the Fish & Wildlife Service, the U.S. Forest Service, the Bureau of Land Management, the Bureau of Reclamation, the Army Engineers or the Tennessee Valley Authority.

Campground hosting — You can camp free for a month or more at a national park if you volunteer to be a campground host. The National Park Service looks for retired people who are knowledgeable campers with their own RVs for those jobs. That means greeting campers, assigning spaces if needed and policing the campground — the kind of work campground managers do. Some who've tried it say it's too much work — others love it, saying it leaves most of their time free for fishing, hiking and day-touring. For details on campground hosting and other volunteer jobs in U.S. parks and forests, visit a park service office or send $3 for the booklet *Helping Out in the Outdoors* to American Hiking Society, 1015 31st St. N.W., Washington, DC 20007.

IN SUMMARY:

— A vast majority of RVers are 49ers-plus.
— If you're a beginning RVer, rent before you buy.
— When you're shopping for an RV, attend the shows and read a good RV magazine.
— To be a camping insider, join an RV club.
— If you don't like meeting people, RVing may not be for you.
— RVers find more unusual places than most travelers.

Travel Tool

★ ★ ★

HOW TO FIND OUT MORE ABOUT RVING

For more information on RVing and camping write these major industry sources:

Good Sam Club, P.O. Box 500, Agoura, CA 91301 ☎ (800/423-5061, in California 800/382-3455).

Kampgrounds of America, P.O. Box 30558, Billings, MT 59114, ☎ (406/248-7444).

National Park Service, Consumer Information Service, P.O. Box 100, Pueblo, CO 81002.

Recreation Vehicle Industry Assn., P.O. Box 2999, Reston, VA 22090, ☎ (703/620-6003).

Major camping directories are:

AAA CampBooks (for each region) (available only to members at American Automobile Association offices in every state).

KOA Directory, Road Atlas and Camping Guide (Kampgrounds of America, Inc., P.O. Box 30558, Billings, MT 59114, and at KOA Kampgrounds).

The National Parks: Camping Guide (Government Printing Office, Washington, DC 20402, #024-005-01028-9).

Rand McNally's Campground & Trailer Park Guide (Rand McNally & Co., 8255 N. Central Park Ave., Skokie, IL 60076, and at bookstores).

Trailer Life's RV Campground and Services Directory (TL Enterprises, 29901 Agoura Rd., Agoura, CA 81301).

Wheeler's RV Resort & Campground Guide (Print Media Services, Ltd., 1521 Jarvis Ave., Elk Grove Village, IL 60007).

Woodall's Campground Directories (Woodall's, 100 Corporate N., Suite 100, Bannock Burn, IL 60015-1255 and at bookstores).

Good books on RVing are:

Home is Where You Park It by Kay Peterson. ($9.45, RoVing Press, Box 2870, Estes Park, CO 80517).

Living in a Motorhome by Laura Wolfe. ($7.45, Woodsong Graphics, Inc., P.O. Box 238, New Hope, PA 18938).

RV Owners Operation & Maintenance Manual. ($6.70, Intertec Publishing Corp., Technical Publications Div., P.O. Box 12901, Overland Park, KS 66212).

Who's Who in RV Rentals ($4.75, Recreation Vehicle Rental Association, 3251 Old Lee Hwy., Ste 500, Fairfax, VA 22030).

Living in Style — The RV Way. ($1.75., Recreation Vehicle Industry Association, P.O. Box 2999, Reston, VA 22090).

Trailer Life's RV Buyer's Guide. ($4.95, TL Enterprises, Inc., 29901 Agoura Rd., Agoura, CA 91301).

Woodall's RV Buyer's Guide. ($5.70, Woodall Publishing Co., 100 Corporate N., Suite 100, Bannock Burn, IL 60015-125511 N. Skokie Hwy., Lake Bluff, IL 60044).

The leading RV magazine is:

Trailer Life, $18/year, P.O. Box 55793, Boulder, CO 80322-5793.

NOTES

CHAPTER 12

BY BUS

Lagniappe: Test of a Successful Tour

Like other Americans, we had never spent much time riding tour buses until we journeyed to Europe for the first time. We believed a bus or motorcoach trip meant confinement or regimentation. And we weren't sure we would like the people we'd be traveling with.

But there we rode buses through the Black Forest, into the Dutch countryside, to France's Fontainebleau and to Shakespeare's Stratford. Enroute we snoozed, talked, sang, read or wrote postcards, arriving at the doorstep of our destination rested and without getting lost.

As a result, like other travelers, we discovered that a motorcoach trip can be the very best way to see an area without hassle or being surprised by high prices.

We've also found that trips organized around our special interests of photography or winetasting are ideal for packaged motorcoach trips.

We can't think of a better way to locate tickets to leading theatrical shows, football games or other special events than by joining a tour.

We've discovered the fun of making — and keeping — friends we have met on motorcoach excursions.

And, most surprising to us, we did not feel confined, nor regimented. In fact, having our own mother hen — in the person of the tour escort to deal with hotel desk clerks or to answer our questions — saved our time for traveling instead of having to spend it on logistics.

171

Some of the tour escorts have been priceless. Like the British fellow whose fly stayed unzipped for the entire trip down the Thames to Greenwich — despite repeated quiet words of warning from his male charges. Even though he cared little about his attire, he had his British history and scenery down cold.

Others have been first-rate quarterbacks. Like the Dutch college girl who ran interference at an overbooked country inn to find us welcome featherbeds for the night.

And some escorts started out as friends from home because they organized the tour. But best of all, they were still our friends when we returned home.

The escort provides the happy chemistry for the group — bringing the people together, solving problems quietly as they occur or taking advantage of an unexpected opportunity to see or do something extra for free; an ingredient that we call lagniappe (pronounced lan-yap).

But the real test of a successful motorcoach trip rests in the planning; the work done in advance by the tour operator behind the scenes.

And whether you enjoy the trip is in the fit; is it right for you?

THE CHANGING TOUR IDEA

Tours are no longer built around the idea of "seeing" something. More and more, the prime ingredient of a tour is "doing" something. As a result, a tour may take you snowmobiling in Yellowstone, rafting a river with stops for gourmet meals, shopping in Ireland or exploring the casinos of Europe just as easily as it can take you through the New England countryside as fall changes the color of the leaves.

Many tours now combine transportation. You may spend part of your time on a train, plane or cruiseship — and on a bus or motorcoach.

Motorcoach-tour ideas come from everywhere, including from you and me. Many tours are made to the order of a club or to fill a need. One tour operator creates trips to the Black Hills for grandparents and grandchildren, while another books a seniors dance club on a cruise. No legal idea is off limits.

SORTING OUT THE OPTIONS

But with so many different trips to choose from, how do we sort them out? Here are some tips:

• Look for a reliable company. Avoid the single-person operator unable to carry an errors-and-omissions insurance policy or to be bonded. One quick way to check is to look at the tour literature for the logo of one of the travel or tour associations: National Tour Association, Inc., of Lexington, Kentucky (NTA); United States Tour Operators Association of New York City (USTOA), American Bus Association of Washington, D.C. (ABA), or American Society of Travel Agents (ASTA). For one thing, these associations maintain ethics committees that review consumer complaints against their members. For another, most have consumer-protection plans that incorporate insurance requirements and establish a minimum number of years' experience.

• Read and understand the itinerary offered. Do you just "drive by" Monticello or do you actually visit it? Does the tour cover the things important to you? Match holidays of the countries to be visited with your tour dates to determine if the things you want to see will be open and operating.

• Determine what will be done each day and which items are included in the package cost. How many meals (beverages and desserts, too) are included? Must you eat from a fixed menu or will there be choices? What kinds of hotels will you be staying in and where are they located? (As one tour operator says, "Question the word 'deluxe' — everyone stays at deluxe hotels so the word means nothing.") Are all admission fees, taxes, luggage handling, airport transfers, transportation and the like paid? Will you be charged extra if you want single accommodations?

• Is the tour paced to please you? Will you really be able to see the attraction offered in the time allowed? Is there adequate free time for you to explore on your own or to rest? How far does the bus travel in a single day, and how frequent are the rest stops? Are meals offered at regular intervals? If you're covering long distances, will there be on-bus activities like eating a box lunch, bingo or sing-alongs, or will the tour operator use a plane to shorten the travel time? Fun Bus Luxury Travel of Anaheim,

Calif., has even developed steward service with sandwiches and soft drinks and sometimes shows movies on closed-circuit TV for tours that cover long, no-scenery stretches of highway. Are there too many stairs or too much walking? Does every day require a 6 a.m. wakeup call?

• What are the operating habits of the tour company? Does it fill the bus to capacity or does it allow the uncomfortable back row and seats over the wheels to be empty? Does it rotate seats from day to day to give everyone a chance at different views and to meet other people? How much and what size luggage is permitted before extra charges are levied? What is the size of the group? Would you be more comfortable in a smaller group or prefer the variety available with more people? What is the company's policy on smoking on the bus? Can you get special-diet meals?

• What kind of equipment does the company use? Do the buses have on-board toilets and refrigerators for cold drinks? Are the windows color-corrected to allow photography? Is the bus air-conditioned?

• What kind of escorts will be with you? Will you have a professional escort or will a member of your social group be in charge? If the leader is a friend or neighbor, will the tour operator provide step-on guides to supply the needed expertise at the attractions to be visited?

• What entertainment is offered? Will there be welcoming cocktail parties and farewell banquets? Will you have a celebrity leading the group? If the tour centers on a special interest, will there be lessons or lectures?

• Are there additional benefits available if you do business with one company over another? Some companies, for example, offer frequent-traveler benefits such as discounts on future trips.

• How does Tour A compare with Tour B in price? If the number of attractions included in the two tours are similar, divide the total tour cost by either the number of days or nights to come up with a unit price for each tour.

For example, tour experts estimate a budget tour will cost you $55 to $65 per day, while a mid-range tour can be expected to cost $75-$90/day and a deluxe tour $125/day and up — depending on where you're going and what the value of the dollar is. But $75/day would not go very far in New York City, while $120/day in many Pacific Rim countries would provide all meals, transportation and 5-star hotels.

For the mid-range price of $75/day you could probably expect to receive one lunch or dinner daily, your transportation, guide, driver, overnight accommodation and daily tour. You would have to buy additional meals and pay tips.

READING THE FINE PRINT

If you've almost made your decision, review the fine print, the "conditions" that are listed at the end of the tour description. Evaluate the tour operator's rights and responsibilities — and yours. If you're in doubt as to what happens when there are schedule substitutions, ask before you go. If you feel your travel agent is not comfortable dealing with motorcoach tours, contact the National Tour Association, P.O. Box 3071, Lexington, KY 40596-3071, and ask for a list of tour companies operating in your area.

Considering how far in advance most tours are planned and booked, think about buying a trip-cancellation insurance policy. The few dollars spent can save hundreds if you become ill or are forced to change plans. One tour operator we know includes a $25 per-person-credit toward purchase of cancellation insurance as part of each major tour package.

TOURING THE CONTINENT

As you plan your overseas travels, you'll have many opportunities to include motorcoach adventures. But each company establishes its own clientele and its own methods. For example, Cosmos is proud that it serves the budget travel market; Europabus is a semiofficial motorcoach operator tied in with European railroads. Be sure you read the brochures carefully to understand the differences. Here are some differences you may encounter:

• Few European buses have on-board toilets, but they do make frequent coffee and comfort breaks. One tour operator describes European buses as "not senior-friendly." He explains that the buses are immaculate and offer large viewing windows.

But they also have steep steps that make maneuvering inside the bus more awkward.

• Many continental bus companies limit passengers to a single suitcase and one flightbag-size carry-on.

• Hotels will more likely be European-style tourist-class with private baths — but the hotels will not always be centrally located. When the hotel is located away from the central district, your bus will take you to the promised attractions.

• Meals are more likely to be a breakfast typical of the country in which you're traveling (continental in Europe, heartier fare in England, Scotland and Ireland), and a dinner about half the time — almost never in major cities. When dinner is offered, it is likely to be a fixed menu, sometimes with a choice of entree.

• Even when single supplements are offered, the companies admit they cannot always provide single accommodations with "private facilities." One brochure explains, "Private facilities means private bath or shower and usually but not always a toilet." As an alternative to single accommodations, some European touring companies offer people-matching services. The services have the benefit of providing the same price to everyone. But you're likely to have at least one roommate as a result.

TRAVELING BY BUS

Until now, we've talked about motorcoach tours. And motorcoach tours are conducted with buses. But not all buses are motorcoaches. We're all familiar with the "leave the driving to us" advertising of Greyhound. And in many parts of the world a point-to-point bus such as a Greyhound is the only way to get where you want to go. After all, not every city has an airport or even a depot.

Even if you had other choices of how to get there, you probably wouldn't have nearly as interesting a time. People who travel by bus tend to be real folks who like to see things up close and personal — and get a bargain at the same time. They don't want to fly over or whiz through the countryside without being able to see it.

And just like airplanes, trains and other tourist-oriented people-movers, bus companies are working to get the attention of us senior travelers. Most Greyhound trips taken by those 65 and over are discounted 10 percent.

BUS DEALS FOR 49ERS-PLUS

We mature travelers are the favored customers of the motor-coach operators. Not only do we fill their buses, but we serve as tour organizers for our churches, senior centers and clubs. In addition, more than one tour operator will tell you they prefer to hire gregarious, organized, well-traveled people around age 55 for their tour leaders.

Even with all of these kind words, tour and bus operators prove over and over that they want our business by offering us special bargains.

For example, one tour operator, Mayflower Tours in Downers Grove, Ill. ☎ 312/960-3430, encourages its customers to repeat by offering Mayflower Money. Mayflower Money pays each traveler $5 a day that can be used as a $5-a-day discount on trips taken within a year.

Frontier Travel and Tours of Carson City, Nev. ☎ 800/648-0912, has developed a Frequent Riders Club that includes a free trip as a reward for every eight paid trips. It also sends a newsletter every other month, offers special days when trips are discounted and uses celebrity hosts.

Globus-Gateway and Cosmos offer 10 percent discounts — not to seniors, but on the fares of grandchildren between 8 and 18 who may accompany them.

Greyhound/Trailways gives 10 percent off every trip ticket for people 65 and over. In addition, it offers the Golden Savers Seniors Club. For a $5 membership for people over 55 in seven Western states (California, Nevada, Utah, Arizona, Washington, Oregon, Idaho), you can get 15 percent off any trip that originates in the West. Plans are afoot to expand this offer to other areas.

The moral of these examples is to ask questions when you shop for tours. You may discover come lagniappe.

WHEN THINGS GO WRONG

Generally we found it's easiest — and more fun — to go with the flow when touring. That doesn't mean things can't go wrong. Nor does it mean that all substitutions live up to the original promise.

As good consumers, we try to document the details of a problem. If the tour brochure promises a tour of Honolulu's Iolani Palace but we only drive around the block, then we start by mentioning the problem to the tour director.

If the problem isn't corrected to our satisfaction, there are other steps to take. Immediately on our return, we contact the tour operator to describe what went wrong and spell out what we expect him to do to correct the situation.

Even though many of us will never return to the same destination twice — which means we may not have a chance to completely repair the wrong — we have to be fair and realistic in what we expect the operator to do to make amends.

If the tour operator ignores your complaint, contact the trade association listed on the original tour brochure. And if that doesn't work, you may have to try your state's attorney general or consumer representative to get help.

But what seems to be important is that with the great numbers of seniors setting out to travel on buses, we are in control of the motorcoach industry. We have told the industry where we want to go, what we want to do, what kind of hotels we like to stay in, what food choices there should be, how long we're willing to ride between stops, what kind of equipment we want on the buses and what kind of tour escorts we find acceptable.

And you know what? The people in charge are listening to what we say.

As a result motorcoach trips for seniors are better than ever.

IN SUMMARY:

— Ideas for motorcoach tours come from everywhere, including from you and me.
— The test of a good motorcoach tour is in the operator's planning.

— Understand the details and terms of the tour you're taking.

— Mature travelers are favored customers of motorcoach operators.

Travel Tool
★ ★ ★

WHERE TO WRITE

Here's where to get more information on motorcoaching:

United State Tour Operators Association
211 E. 51st St. #12B, New York, NY 10022.
☎ 212/944-5727.
Ask for *How to Select a Package Tour.*

National Tour Association, Inc.,
546 E. Main St., P.O. Box 3071, Lexington KY 40596-3071.
☎ 606/253-1036; 800/682-8886 (US); 800/828-6999 (Canada).
Ask for *Your Next Vacation Could Be Your Best Ever*, the brochure *Travel Together* and *A Consumer's Guide to National Tour Association Operator Companies, What is the National Tour Association Consumer Protection Plan?*

American Bus Association
1025 Connecticut Avenue, N.W., #308, Washington DC 20036.
☎ 202/293-5890.

Travel Tool
★ ★ ★

THE LANGUAGE OF MOTORCOACHING

Here are some terms you'll need to know when you're shopping for a motorcoach tour:

All-inclusive—Price includes round-trip transportation and land arrangements.

American Plan (AP)—Breakfast, lunch, dinner.

Continental breakfast—Bread or pastries, butter and jam, hot beverage.

Double occupancy rate—Price per person based on two people sharing a room.

Double-room rate—The full price of the room shared by two persons.

Driver-guide—A driver who also describes points of interest.

Escorted—A tour that includes an escort, manager or director who accompanies tour from place to place.

Force majeure—An event that cannot be reasonable anticipated or controlled.

Full board or pension—Breakfast, lunch, dinner.

Half board or demi-pension—Breakfast and either lunch or dinner

Land price—Price for land arrangements only.

High-season supplement—Extra charge for peak season.

Independent—Packaged arrangements for people traveling on their own.

Local host—Tour operator employee who provides assistance in a single city or area.

Modified American Plan (MAP)—Breakfast, dinner.

Pension—A European guesthouse/inn.

Porterage—Baggage handling service not including tips.

Table d'hote—A full-course meal served at a fixed price.

Tour escort/manager/director—Professional who accompanies the group and oversees travel arrangements.

Transfers—Transportation between place you arrive, such as airport, and place you stay, such as hotel.

CHAPTER 13

CRUISING

A Promise of Adventure for 49ers-Plus

For 49ers-plus, cruising is about the best travel value around. Whatever you've learned about cruising aboard TV's *Love Boat*, you don't have to eat five meals a day, disco till dawn, then spend the whole next day touring Acapulco — in fact, cruising can be the most laid-back, relaxed vacation you've ever taken, if you want it that way.

On the other hand, cruising almost always fulfills its promise of adventure: exotic new sights, interesting new friends, tempting new foods — and, yes, romance, even for the 49er-plus.

There's no doubt that cruising is addictive. Studies show that people who cruise once tend to cruise again and again. On the other hand, only 30 percent of the traveling public has ever taken a first cruise, and some studies put that number as low as 5 percent.

The best part of cruising is the prices, which are tumbling at an astounding rate. Each year, worldwide, more people take to cruising, and each year a dozen new ships or more come on-line. Despite this surge in cruising's popularity, there will still be more cabins than people to fill them into the 1990s.

WHERE TO CRUISE

Because almost 90 percent of the earth is covered by water, you can cruise nearly everywhere. Even cruise veterans seldom run out of places to go.

The most common cruise destinations for Americans these days are Alaska, the Caribbean, Mexico. And for mature travelers, add those glorious seven-day Hawaii cruises to the most-popular list — in our opinion, the very best way to see the islands.

What about a Panama Canal passage, an ocean crossing on the QE2 or a Carnival season cruise to South America? You can fly to Tahiti and cruise the South Seas islands, fly to Hong Kong, Bangkok or Singapore to cruise the Orient, or to London, Copenhagen or Oslo for a Scandinavian cruise.

Many take the four-day Greek Island cruises, but other Mediterranean cruises are as numerous as those to the Caribbean: the route of Marco Polo from Venice, the Riviera and the Costa del Sol, around the boot of Italy, to Dubrovnik, to Cairo, to Gibraltar, to Spain and Portugal, to the Holy Land, to the North African ports where pirates waited to plunder.

And who said you had to be on the ocean? There are wonderful little barge canal cruises all over England and Western Europe, especially France. And grand ones on the Rhine and the Danube rivers. You can cruise various portions of the Nile aboard comfortable hotel boats, take ocean-going vessels more than a thousand miles up the Amazon or far into the St. Lawrence, or sail on a steamboat to the upper reaches of the Mississippi.

That's just a start — some ideas to get your thinking moving.

WAYS TO CRUISE

Most cruises, of course, are aboard ocean-going vessels that are designed to carry 600 to 1,500 passengers in comfortable-to-elegant style.

But there are other ways to cruise, too, that 49ers-plus will enjoy:

Freighter cruises — Yes, almost all freighters carry passengers, and they go to far more places than passenger ships do, at comparable prices. These are for cruising veterans who want a more leisurely pace and don't need a cruise director to tell them what to see. Freighter cruises last for months, going from port to obscure port, stopping a few days to load or drop cargo (which gives you touring time ashore), sometimes switching schedules or making surprise stops. These are not your typical slow boats to China. Rather, modern freighters — many of them container ships — are designed to carry up to 80 passengers quite comfortably, with spacious quarters, superb food usually in the officer's mess and no fixed schedule. Freighter cruising is a subculture on which you have to get hooked — but those who do it say they'll never travel any other way. You can often book freighter cruises direct with the line's agent, and there are two or three travel agencies that specialize in freighter cruises. To locate them, subscribe to Lee Pledger's *Freighter Travel News* ($18 for 12 monthly issues), P.O. Box 12693, Salem, OR 97309.

Barge cruises — Elegant hotel barges that carry, at most, 24 passengers (and as few as eight) ply the spiderweb canal system of England and the narrow rivers of France and other European countries. You'll sleep and eat aboard these boats as the personal guests of the captain and his mate. Hop off when you want and help pull the boat, ride a bike to a nearby chateau or just walk along the bank; then come back aboard for a gourmet dinner (aren't all dinners in France gourmet?) and a bottle of wine or two. And what could be more idyllic (or decadent) than cruising through Burgundy at 12 miles a day during the grape harvest, or reaching up the Avon during an English summer? For a catalog, call Floating Through Europe toll-free at ☎ 800/221-3140, or ask your travel agent.

River cruises — The world's two greatest waterways host the two most popular river cruises — albeit, on different continents and on quite dissimilar vessels. The great, modern motorships of the KD German Rhine Line course that river like white dolphins, from Basel in Switzerland to the seaport of Amsterdam in Holland. You'll see castles perched atop the gorges of the Rhine, and grapes suffering in vineyards that climb straight up mountainsides. You'll cruise during the day and lay in to a river village overnight so as not to miss any of the scenery. On shore excursions, often you'll go ashore at one village, tour some inland site while the ship moves on and pick it up at the next town. For brochures and schedules, write Rhine Cruise Agency, 170 Hamilton Ave., White Plains, NY 10601 ☎ (toll-free 800/346-6525 in the eastern U.S., 800/858-8587 in the West).

When you step aboard the lavish Delta Queen or Mississippi Queen steamboats, cruising from New Orleans as far north as St.

Paul, Minn., or Pittsburgh on the Ohio River, you'll step back in time. You'll pass antebellum homesteads and visit historic towns that helped to shape the nation. These cruises are run by the Delta Queen Steamboat Co., No. 30 Robin Street Wharf, New Orleans, LA 70130 ☎ toll-free 800/543-1949.

A CRUISE PRIMER

Here are some common things that are part of almost every cruise experience:

Baggage — A porter will take custody of your bags on the dock. Later, they'll appear in your stateroom automatically — almost always. But sometimes it's a couple of hours after the ship sails. If you're nervous about that kind of thing, as we are, and if you pack light, as we do, you may want to carry the bags aboard yourself.

Lifeboat drill — Everybody is required to get into these wonderfully funny orange balloon jackets and stand around at exact spots on deck while a ship's officer counts heads and tells you what would happen should the ship start sinking. It looks like a convention of Michelin men; the ship's photographer pops pictures of all the roly-polies, and all have a great time.

Eating — You get at least five or six shots at it every day. Breakfast is buffet-style on the fantail, or served to you in the main dining room. Same for lunch. There are snacks at mid-morning and mid-afternoon. There are usually two dinner seatings around 6 p.m. And at midnight there's a buffet. Ships, of course, specialize in the cuisine of their countries. In addition, on most ships you can request kosher meals when you book your cruise, as well as vegetarian meals, salt-free meals and other kinds of diet meals. There's always a wine list. You'll select dinner seating when you board the ship. You'll usually have a choice of table for two, four, six or eight, then you'll stay with the same tablemates throughout the cruise. We find six makes for the best conversation.

Morning laps — We've never been on a cruise ship that didn't have somebody leading a mile of early morning laps — jogging or walking — around the decks.

Dress — Take the clothes you're comfortable in. Dress is casual, especially on the shorter cruises — sometimes too casual.

It always bothers us in the evening to see blue jeans in the dining room — but that is often permitted. On classier, higher-priced cruises like Sitmar's and Cunard's, men will need a tux or dinner jacket, and women a gown. Usually, one dress-up outfit will do — jacket and tie for men, heels and a dressier pants-suit or dress for women — for the captain's reception and formal night in the dining room. Otherwise, you can spend all day around decks in swimsuit or shorts. Bring clothes that are breezy and loose-fitting, a good pair of walking shoes and a sun-hat for shore trips. For evenings at sea bring a sweater, even in the summer. If a costume night is scheduled, you can usually get one aboard ship.

Photographer — The ubiquitous ship's photographer will snap you doing almost anything — in fact, you can't stop him. He'll snap you coming aboard, at the lifeboat drill, at dinner, with the captain, going on tour, wearing your silly sun-hat, whatever. Your mug will be posted somewhere on the ship at least half-a-dozen times during the cruise — and every photo is for sale.

Other facilities — Most cruise ships come with barber and hairdresser, exercise facilities, duty-free gift shop, massage treatments, radio room for ship-shore calls, doctor, disco, movie theater, kids' game arcade and casino. There are plenty of small lounges and nooks — both indoors and out — for just sitting around and reading or snoozing. We've often wondered, though, why news rarely seems to get aboard — you may see some TV, but you usually have to get newspapers ashore.

Captain's reception — There's one on every cruise . . . the only time most passengers get to see the skipper. Dress to the scuppers for this one. They'll feed you through the reception line, take your photo with the captain and hand you a glass of champagne. Afterward, the captain will say a few kind words and introduce his officers. The whole thing takes less than an hour — attendance is optional, but we always think it's nice to meet the fellow who drives the ship.

Shore tours — At every stop you can take a choice of tours that will start at the dock and get you back before the ship sails. The cruise director's staff briefs you on shore tours early in the cruise, so you know exactly what each one involves. Or you can have the cruise director arrange to have a rented car waiting at the dock for you so you can tour on your own.

Seasickness — "A cruiseship," said one first-time passenger, "is like a giant waterbed." These are big ships, usually sailing relatively calm seas; the motions are gentle. And most modern ships are equipped with stabilizers, which eliminate about two-thirds of the natural motion — if you think you'll have a problem, select a ship with stabilizers. We find the roll of the ship actually helps put us to sleep at night. Nevertheless, a few passengers always end up woozy the first night out. Dramamine works, but the new transderm scops — "ear patches" that release small doses of medicine throughout the cruise — work better. Though you can't get them ashore except by prescription, on most ships the purser passes out free patches like they were lollipops. Other advice: take an inside cabin on the centerline deep in the ship (the point which moves the least). Nowadays, few passengers return seasick — and those few don't usually return to sea.

Tipping — Most ships post a "suggested" tipping schedule that includes everyone from the room steward to the busboy. The custom is that on the last night, you trip around like the good fairy handing out mysterious envelopes to those who've treated you well. Keep at least $50-$70 cash for tips — or you can cash a check at the purser's desk.

Passports — If your cruise takes you outside American waters, you may need some proof of citizenship when you go ashore. A passport is always the best one. If you don't have a passport, take your birth certificate or voter registration card.

Customs — Whenever you come from a foreign port, you have to return through U.S. customs. You'll get a thorough briefing from ship's staff before you dock. It's hassle-free — customs officers usually take your word for what you've bought, and rarely go through your bags. Nevertheless, it takes time — allow at least two hours after docking in the United States before you're permitted to make shore connections. Don't even try to cut it close — with an 8 a.m. docking in Los Angeles, for instance, you'd miss a 10:30 flight from LAX, which is an hour's drive from the port.

THE STARTER CRUISE

For mature travelers who've never cruised before, we feel the ideal first cruise is a three- or four-day trip from one of the major U.S. ports into the Caribbean or along the Baja California coast.

These short starter cruises share most of the advantages of longer, more traditional voyages: you don't have to pack and unpack at each new destination; you're pampered from start to finish, and there are few surprises that will bust your budget. You are at sea long enough to learn how cruising is done, sample most of its customs and find out whether cruising is for you.

The popular "cruises to nowhere" or one-day trips out the Florida ports to Freeport, Bahamas, and back, are too short to give you that kind of complete cruise experience; yet, if you find you don't like ocean cruising, you are not committed to another week or 10 days, nor have you spent a bundle. The cost of a short cruise can be less than $100 a day — and that includes all meals, and often airfare. The only extras will be shore tours, gifts, your bar bill and tips — all optional and not really necessary, except for the tips.

The main reason they've never taken a cruise, some other mature travelers tell us, is the problem of getting started — overcoming natural fears and getting on board for the first time. To lure the 70 percent who have never cruised, more steamship companies are adding short cruises to their itineraries.

That seems to be working. Aboard Admiral Cruise Lines' SS Azure Seas, making three- and four-day cruises out of Los Angeles, Capt. Dimitrios Flokos told us that 60 percent of his passengers invariably are first-time cruisers. And most of those eventually return to the sea once, twice, or even more often. Many have become regulars on Azure Seas cruises, Flokos said. One woman had logged 150 trips on the Azure Seas — but many more graduate to longer, more luxurious cruises.

Azure Seas has been cruising out of Los Angeles since 1980. In 1988, Norwegian Cruise Lines' Southward joined the trade. Both ships sail to Santa Catalina Island off the California Coast, then down to Ensenada, Mexico, and return to L.A. San Diego is an added stop on four-day cruises. There are similar cruises out of Miami. Other regularly scheduled short cruises now leave from the Florida ports of Tampa, Port Canaveral and Port

Everglades. A list of these starter cruises is at the end of this chapter.

Charlanne F. Herring, in her informative *Cruise Answer Book*, lists the dozen or more ships making regular short cruises as "fun" ships, which she defines as featuring "non-stop activity, party atmosphere, usually appealing to younger passengers." Yes, the companies currently staging these short cruises are trying to lure young adults aboard, figuring after their first cruise, they'll be lifetime cruise addicts. But, ironically, they're really luring lots of 49ers-plus.

On our recent Azure Seas voyage, almost half the passengers clearly were 49ers-plus. And the ship's Capt. Flokos confirmed that's a usual mix. "Many retired people like to take a few days off and sail around," Flokos told us. "Many of our regular passengers are retired people." Of course — we're the ones who have the time to take these trips, especially the midweek ones. The youngsters still have to work.

As for "non-stop activity," it's true. As the cruise director explained the first night, "We'll try to give you the whole cruise experience you'd get on a 10-day cruise — but just in four days." That doesn't mean you have to take part in everything — the casino games, the movies, the tours, the singalongs, the singles' mix 'n' mingles, the disco, the morning laps, the exercise classes, the arts and crafts, the dance classes, the daily bingo, the cabaret shows, the bridge tours, the backgammon tournament, the passenger talent show, the shuffleboard tournament, the Grandmothers Get-Together and Afternoon Tea or the white-elephant auction. As on any cruise, shipboard activities are non-stop every day to give passengers a choice of things to do. But the only activity you have to take part in is the lifeboat drill. After that, you can loaf away the whole cruise like a toad on a warm boulder.

The whole object of cruising, in fact, is to relax. As the woman was telling her friend in the Azure Seas dinner line after our day on Catalina: "No tour today. I just rolled up in my blankie and went out on deck and catnapped. And it was wonderful."

THE LOW COST OF CRUISING

In the cruise business, any rate under $150 a day per person is a true bargain. But nowadays you can cruise to the Caribbean, to Mexico and even to Alaska for little more than $100 a day, sometimes less — and that includes airfare.

A five-day Caribbean cruise on Bermuda Star Line's SS Veracruz, for example, runs $299 to $469. Day-cruises from Florida to Freeport in the Bahamas cost seniors as little as $69.

Though most cruiselines will be keeping prices the same or raising them only slightly, nobody will be buying cruises at the posted prices, according to the authoritative *Travel Weekly*.

Cruise discounts come in lots of disguises:

If you book your cruise early — say, three months or more, almost all cruiselines offer a few hundred dollars off the price. If you book late, last-minute travel agencies will get you a cut-rate deal on the cruise you want (see Chapter 3, Your Friend, the Travel Agent). If you book in-between, discount agencies will help you out.

In addition, the few cruiselines unwilling to cut their prices will throw in extras — free or low-cost air supplements, free hotel rooms before or after your cruise, stateroom upgrades, spending certificates to use aboard ship. Some have stretched their cruises — eight days for the price of seven, for example, or Glacier Bay cruises that now go beyond Anchorage. And some operators, like Holland America and Princess Tours, add a land package to their Anchorage cruises — train trips past Mt. McKinley to Fairbanks.

Shop the travel section of your Sunday newspaper for cruise deals. And catch the flavor of the ads. Most cruiselines forbid discounters from advertising in terms of dollars. Look for catchwords like "group discount," or for discounts stated as percentages off regular rates, rather than dollars off.

But don't try to find a bargain by yourself. Because of the bewildering number of cruises, you should work through a travel agent to find the best values for the place you want to cruise to. There are retail travel agents, as well as discounters, who specialize only in cruises.

And make sure your travel agent has worked aggressively to find you the best price on the cruise you want to take. In any case, do not pay the advertised price for a cruise unless there are lots of offsetting extras.

POSITIONING CRUISES

There are some things that only your travel agent — or maybe your Sunday travel section — can tell you.

Positioning cruises are one-shot voyages planned to get a ship from an old home port to a new one. For example, a Seattle-based ship that sails weekly to Glacier Bay in the summer is repositioned to Miami for weekly Caribbean cruises in the winter. Positioning cruises are a time for crew rotation, for chefs to experiment with new menu items, for lounge entertainers to try out new numbers. Everything takes on a new freshness during such a voyage.

And it will be a lovely cruise — perhaps two or three weeks — with stops to pick up and drop off passengers in San Francisco, Los Angeles, Acapulco or other Mexican Riviera ports, then a passage through the Panama Canal. There'll be Caribbean ports new to many crewmen, and lots of interaction between crew and passengers as both explore.

They'll fly you to Seattle and fly you home from Miami. And the cost will be one-half to two-thirds of what you'd normally pay for such a cruise. Example: when Royal Cruise Lines repositioned Crown Odyssey from San Juan, P.R., to Lisbon, you could have gotten on the 13-day cruise for as little as $1,400 (with an early-booking discount) — and that included round-trip airfare to U.S. gateways and three nights at a Lisbon hotel.

The rates are cheap because cruiselines don't put a lot of advertising or promotion effort into positioning cruises, and yet there have to be passengers to make the cruise work. They are great for retirees, who have the time to take a longer cruise and the flexibility to plan well in advance and, thus, take advantage of early-booking discounts.

Usually, only your travel agent knows when all of the positioning cruises are scheduled, and which ones offer deeply discounted early-booking rates.

Just tell your agent you're in the market for such a cruise, and to alert you whenever a good one comes up on the computer.

DEALS AT SEA FOR 49ERS-PLUS

Because half or more of those who cruise are 49ers-plus, senior-citizen discounts are rare at sea, and most of those offered are either one-time deals or just for club members.

AARP offers its members cruises at rates you probably couldn't get through a retail travel agency (though a discounter might match them), as do clubs like Mature Outlook, Good Sam and AAA. Grand Circle Travel and Saga Holidays, packaging trips exclusively for 49ers-plus, occasionally offer cruises at attractive prices — up to 30 percent off — to those on their mailing lists (see Chapter 2, The Savvy Senior, for addresses).

The only long-running deal for seniors at sea that we know of is the result of a rate war in south Florida between SeaEscape, Dolphin Cruise Lines, Premier Cruise Lines and Discovery Cruises. These lines give seniors 10 percent or more off most of their cruises.

Ships leave Miami, Fort Lauderdale or Port Everglades daily for one-day "cruises to nowhere" and to Freeport in the Bahamas, and for overnighters to Freeport. Regular rates range from $39 to $99 a day, including meals aboard ship — then take off 10 percent if you're over 55 or carry an AARP card. Discovery gives seniors $10 off all cruises, and the price for that one-day Bahamas cruise is as low as $39 to start with — that's a 25 percent discount.

Even better, Premier Cruise Lines gives seniors 10 percent off on all its cruises, including three- and four-day starter cruises to the Caribbean, some of which are combined with free Disney World packages.

Book these cruises through your travel agent.

If you're visiting Florida, these cruises make a nice short side-trip into a different world than the one you see on the road. If you live there, they make a low-cost day's outing and a chance to meet new people in a party atmosphere.

CRUISE HOSTS

Among the most innovative cruise deals for 49ers-plus are Royal Cruise Lines' Host and Commander's Club programs.

Simply put, congenial, sophisticated guys 50 and older can get free cruises if they'll spend their time escorting congenial single gals 50 and older at shipboard activities. RCL's research found that, while many women go on cruises without male escorts, it's harder when you're over 49 to find single male companions on board ship.

Hosts on RCL's luxury ships Golden Odyssey and Crown Odyssey, which cruise over most of the world's oceans, serve as dancing, dining and card-playing partners for women traveling alone. They have liberal bar tabs, go with groups on shore trips, attend cocktail parties and take part in other ship's social activities.

There is usually a Host for every 10 single women booked on a cruise. Hosts are under strict orders to mingle, with no favoritism toward any one passenger or group. Romantic relationships are out. RCL says it screens Host candidates thoroughly for "a combination of general congeniality, respectability, travel experience and enthusiasm for nightly dancing." Most are retired or semi-retired professional men, according to an RCL spokesman.

To get more information on becoming a Host, write Host Program, Royal Cruise Line, One Maritime Plaza, 14th Floor, San Francisco, CA 94111.

The Commander's Club is the same kind of program to encourage solo males to take cruises — except you can be any age, you pay $5 a year, and you get only 20 percent discounts on selected cruises and shore packages, $100 bar credit and $50-a-day single stateroom supplement.

But Commanders Clubbers can have all the romance they want.

IN SUMMARY:

— Cruising is one of the best travel values for 49ers-plus.
— Most popular cruise destinations for seniors are Alaska, Hawaii, the Caribbean and Mexico.
— First-timers can choose a shorter voyage to get the flavor of cruising.
— Though cruise prices are coming down, discounts just for seniors are fairly rare at sea.

Travel Tool

BOOKS ON CRUISING

Here are some books on cruises that will help the first-time traveler or the veteran. All are available in book stores:

The Cruise Answer Book: A Comprehensive Guide to the Ships and Ports of North America by Charlanne F. Herring ($9.95. Mills & Sanderson, publisher). Basic cruise lore, tips for first-time cruisers as well as veterans. Second section describes ships, ports of call, cruise rates, shore excursions available for the most popular cruising areas.

Fielding's Worldwide Guide to Cruises by Antoinette DeLand ($12.95. William Morrow & Co., publisher). Lists all major cruise lines, their addresses and histories. Describes major destinations around the world, and more than 100 cruise ships.

Caribbean Ports of Call by Kay Showker ($14.95. The Globe Pequot Press, publisher). How to make the most of a vacation at sea in a limited time. Describes Caribbean ports, and profiles cruise lines and ships plying the Caribbean.

CLIA Question and Answer Booklet. A cruising primer. Send a stamped, addressed envelope with 45¢ postage to Cruise Lines International Association, 500 Fifth Ave., Ste. 1407, New York, NY 10110.

Travel Tool

STARTER CRUISES

Here are ships making three- and four-day starter cruises from U.S. Ports:

From Los Angeles:

Azure Seas — Every Monday & Friday to San Diego (Monday departures only), Catalina, Ensenada. 734 passengers.

Stabilizers. No handicap facilities. 734 passengers. $455-$975. (Admiral Cruises).

Southward — Every Monday & Friday to San Diego (Monday departures only), Catalina, Ensenada. 730 passengers. Stabilizers. Handicap facilities. $345-$885. (Norwegian Cruise Line).

From Miami:

Emerald Seas — Every Monday & Friday to Freeport (Mondays only), Nassau, Little Stirrup Cay. 790 passengers. No stabilizers. Handicap facilities. $395-$1,065. (Admiral Cruises).

Carnivale — Every Monday & Friday to Freeport (Mondays only), Nassau. 950 passengers. Stabilizers. No handicap facilities. $375-$1,025. (Carnival Cruise Lines).

Dolphin IV — Every Monday & Friday to Freeport (Mondays only), Nassau, Dolphin Cove. 730 passengers. Stabilizers. No handicap facilities. $425-$915. (Dolphin Cruise Line).

Sunward II — Every Monday & Friday to Freeport (Mondays only), Nassau, Bahamas out-island. 686 passengers. Stabilizers. Handicap facilities. $345-$845. (Norwegian Cruise Line).

From Port Everglades:

Mardi Gras — Every Thursday & Sunday to Freeport (Sundays only), Nassau. 906 passengers. Stabilizers. No handicap facilities. $375-$1,025. (Carnival Cruise Lines).

From Port Canaveral:

Star/Ship Oceanic — Every Monday & Friday to Nassau, Bahamas out-island. Can be combined with Disney package. 1,100 passengers. Stabilizers. Handicap facilities. $355-$1,055. (Premier Cruise Lines).

Star/Ship Majestic — Every Thursday and Sunday to the Abacos, the Bahamas' "family islands. Can be combined with Disney package. 750 passengers. Stabilizers, handicap facilities. $395-$960. (Premier Cruise Lines).

SHORTER SHORT CRUISES

While these trips are too short to provide a complete cruising experience, you can get a taste of the sea aboard these mini-cruises:

Two-day cruises — Chandris' Britanis, every Friday Miami-Nassau (summers only), $189-$370.

One-day cruises — SeaEscape's Scandinavian Star, daily Miami-Freeport, seniors' fare $79. Chandris' Amerikanis, every Saturday New York cruise to nowhere, overnight (summers only), $119-$199. SeaEscape's Scandinavian Sun, Sun.-Fri. Port Everglades-Freeport-Fort Lauderdale, seniors' fare $79. SeaEscape's Scandinavian Sky, Port Canaveral daily cruise to nowhere, $79 (10 percent seniors' discount). Crown's Viking Princess, Wed., Fri., Sun. Palm Beach cruise to nowhere, $59; Mon., Tues., Thurs., Sat. Palm Beach-Freeport, $79. SeaEscape Scandinavian Saga, St. Petersburg daily cruise to nowhere, $79.

NOTES

CHAPTER 14

TRAINS

| For Mature Travelers, They Can Be Time Machines |

I t's not so important where you go on a train — it's how you get there that's the joy. For mature travelers, a train can be a time machine — a journey into the not-too-distant past.

True, most of America's great trains are gone — sleek luxury rides like the Twentieth Century Limited, the swift Northwestern 400, the Super Chiefs. Jetliners, which cut days off the long journey from east to west and at prices not too much higher, almost put America's trains out of business.

But now Amtrak is trying hard to restore the ambience of those great trains, with their elegant diners and club cars and superb service, and on western routes especially, seems to be making it work.

Amtrak runs trains like the Coast Starlight from Seattle to Los Angeles and the California Zephyr along the old Union Pacific route from Chicago to San Francisco that are truly land cruises, with some of the best mountainscapes in America that you simply can't glimpse from an automobile. And more and more packagers, like American Zephyr, are creating tours that showcase trips on the Amtrak — big band weekends, trips from Washington to Colonial Williamsburg, shopping trips to New York, one-day murder-mystery trips and the like. Book any of these through your travel agent, or contact American Zephyr Tours at 1 W. 37th St. 8th floor, New York, NY 10018 ☎ phone 212/764-6266.

In Europe, where distances are shorter and it often takes no longer to go by train than by plane, railroads are still the preferred way to travel. The trains we've seen in Europe are modern, clean and about the most convenient way to get from City A to City B that we know of. The fares are cheap and departures are frequent.

And for visitors from America, the Europeans have found ways to make train travel even more desirable, with special passes and senior-citizen discounts.

ALL ABOARD THE AMTRAK

Our attorney, a nostalgia buff, once took his young daughter on the Amtrak from Reno over the snowy Sierra passes to Davis, Calif., which he computed as the halfway point on the journey to San Francisco. An hour later, they climbed aboard the Amtrak going the other direction back home to Reno.

He just wanted her to see what a train ride was like before the trains disappeared.

Later, we took the trip ourselves, just to get away for a day. And it was a wonderfully refreshing break, much like the old days of train travel.

The trains, of course, are not disappearing in America — far from it. And the Amtrak is relaying its claim as a legitimate way to travel — especially for pleasure travelers — whether on short journeys or longer ones.

You can spend weeks aboard the train seeing different parts of America — and at a cost the airlines can't begin to match. Amtrak, clearly, wants America's vacation business.

For snowbirds who don't look forward to a long drive, Amtrak runs auto trains from Virginia to Florida and back—and off-season one-way rates (northbound trains in the fall, southbound trains in the spring) are low.

To lure vacationers off planes, Amtrak's All Aboard America Fares permit travelers to see the whole country for as little as $299.

And everywhere the Amtrak goes — from major cities, to the Adirondacks to Yosemite Park — it has arranged side-trip packages and escorted tours for those who want to get off the train and linger awhile.

Amtrak's land-cruiser trains — those that make longer journeys — are self-contained, with a range of sleeping compart-

198

ments and complete meal service. You can leave your day-coach seat, stretch your legs around the train or ride in Vistadome cars for better views of the country you're passing through. You can have a drink, play cards — or just lounge — in the lounge car. Just as in the old days, smiling porters roam the train to serve you drinks, make up your berth or take care of any other service you need. Truly, it's a relaxing way to travel.

As a generalization, travel on the Amtrak costs about half as much as air travel. Amtrak has a complicated fare structure, including a 25 percent senior discount on coach fares and seasonal specials. But it all boils down to three simple "All Aboard America Fares" that are far below most of Amtrak's other promotional fares.

Here's an example: to fly from New York to Miami costs $450 (round-trip coach), and the airlines' lowest promotional fare is $238 (with all kinds of early-purchase restrictions and penalties). The round-trip train fare is $372, with the senior discount bringing it to $279. But if you're traveling on Amtrak's All Aboard America pass, the round-trip is only $149-$159, and you can take a side trip to boot. Of course, a sleeper compartment will be extra.

Never mind the senior discount: Amtrak does not offer any senior discount on All Aboard America fares — but even so, they're a bargain. Here's how the passes work:

The country is divided into three regions — East, Midwest (starting at Indianapolis and New Orleans) and West (starting at Denver, Albuquerque and El Paso). You can visit within one region for $159, two regions for $239 and three regions for $299. You can take 45 days to make your trip, stop off anywhere and visit any three cities along your route.

For $299, you could start out in Boston, for example, and travel to Chicago; change trains for the Twin Cities and Seattle; take the Coast Starlight down through San Francisco to Los Angeles; change again for Phoenix, San Antonio, Houston and New Orleans; and travel back up through Dixie to Washington and home through the Northeast Corridor to Boston. And you could stop off at any three cities along your route, perhaps even taking one of Amtrak's escorted tour packages.

That, in our view, is a great way to see all of America — with all the leisure of cruising, without the hassle of driving, without the expense of air travel. But remember that All Aboard trips on the Amtrak are "ticketed" — that is planned in advance — unlike Eurail trips where you can just hop aboard on a vacation trip as you fancy.

On the other hand, using the Amtrak just to get from city to city won't save you much compared with airfare, especially for short distances, and it can take more time than driving would.

You can get information on Amtrak tours, fares and timetables at any Amtrak station, from your travel agent or from Amtrak Distribution Center, P.O. Box 7717, Itasca, IL 60143; ☎ toll-free 800/872-7245.

TRAIN TRAVEL TIPS

Of course, you have to pack differently if you're taking a long train trip. Baggage that you check through you won't see until journey's end. So you'll need to pack an overnighter to keep with you. In addition to toiletries, medication and the like, put in pajamas, slippers and a change or two of clothing.

That's true whether you plan to spend nights in the comfortable, reclining seat that comes with your Amtrak coach fare, or in a sleeping compartment. Long-distance coach sections on Amtrak have large dressing rooms where you can change your clothes for nighttime. On coaches, you'll get a pillow but no blanket.

Take along a sweater or jacket, whether it's winter or summer, in case the air conditioning gets too cold or the heater isn't working. Dress aboard trains is much less formal than it used to be — low-heeled shoes and slacks for women, slacks and a sports shirt or sports jacket for men.

Count on carrying your own bags through the station to the baggage department — redcaps, though still available at larger stations, are becoming scarcer, though you can often get a baggage cart. On most European trains, you can keep your baggage with you. As at airports, lock your bags and put luggage tags on each one, whether or not you check them through.

Whenever you leave your seat for the dining car or lounge, take your valuables with you. Don't leave money or other valuables in coat or jacket pockets above your seats.

As on airplanes, you can get special diet meals — vegetarian or kosher, for example — by making arrangements with Amtrak 72 hours in advance.

OTHER NORTH AMERICAN TRAINS

Canada has its own rail system, called Via Rail. The continent's longest rail trip is on Via Rail's Canadian, a 3,639-mile run from Halifax to Vancouver that takes four days. Of course, you can limit your trip to the scenic parts, from Vancouver to Calgary through the Canadian Rockies, or up the St. Lawrence between Montreal and Nova Scotia.

In the summer, Via Rail trains run north-south into Hudson Bay country and into the Yukon.

Via Rail gives travelers 65 and over one-third off its posted fares. For information, rates, timetables, tours and route maps, call Via Rail toll free at ☎ 800/665-0200. A good book describing some of the best trips on Via Rail is Bill Coo's *Scenic Rail Guide to Western Canada*. For a copy, send $10 to Bradt Enterprises, Inc., 95 Harvey St., Cambridge, MA 02140.

Farther north, the Alaska State Railway runs passenger trains, with Vistadomes and conductors in each car who talk about points of interest, from Seward and Anchorage through Denali National Park to Fairbanks, Alaska — some of the best scenery and wildlife viewing in North America. The one-day trip costs less than $100 one-way, but there are no senior citizen discounts. The trains run from late May to mid-September.

At least two tour companies piggyback their own luxury cars on the train, and offer overnight stops in the park, plus some side trips. You can also take the train as part of an Alaska cruise on Princess Tours and Holland America Lines. Train-only tours range from $279 a person on Princess Tours' two-day Midnight Sun Express tour, to $689 for Westours' McKinley Explorer five-day tours. For information and reservations, call the Alaska State Railway ☎ toll-free at 800/544-0552; Princess Tours at ☎ 800/835-8907; or Gray Line of Alaska (for Holland America's McKinley Explorer) at ☎ 800/544-2206.

TRAINS IN EUROPE

If you're traveling on your own and visiting several cities in Europe, the trains are the best way to go. The trains go everywhere, and unlike major airports, railroad depots are usually in the heart of town and convenient to hotels. Equipment and service are at least as good as the Amtrak's — more often, better. And the cost can be surprisingly low.

Though most European rail systems have senior-citizen passes or discounts off regular fares (see table at the end of this chapter), most American travelers in Europe are better off with a Eurailpass. After you buy one of these, you can travel for a fixed period of time anywhere in Western Europe, except Great Britain, — plus Hungary. You can travel on any train, including the fast trains, except the privately operated luxury trains like the Orient Express. Eurailpasses are just for foreign tourists — they're not sold in Europe. Buy them in the United States and Canada from your travel agent or direct from Eurail. Write for the free timetable, *Through Europe by Train*, a Eurail map and brochure to CIT Tours, 666 Fifth Ave., New York, NY 10103. Current costs are $320 for a 15-day pass, $398 for 21 days and $498 for a month. Two-month and three-month passes are also available.

A BritRail Pass is good anywhere in Great Britain, except Northern Ireland. BritRail Passes cost slightly less than Eurail and are sold at British Rail Offices as well as travel agencies in North America and the European continent — but not in Great Britain.

You'll save the most money on a Eurail Pass if you're traveling frequently in several countries, especially the high-fare countries of northern Europe. If you're traveling only in one or two countries, check out other passes and senior discounts offered by their national rail systems. You have to buy these at the station — your travel agent can't help you. If you're planning an extended stay — more than three months — the individual passes with their senior discounts are also better deals.

TIPS ON EUROPEAN RAIL TRAVEL

You can make reservations on almost any European train just a few hours before it departs, except possibly in the summer, when trains are jammed. Then you have to plan your train trips well in advance. If you're worried about a language problem, ask the concierge at your hotel to make your reservations.

Some European rail cars have center aisles, just like those in North America. Others have compartments that hold up to six people. If you want a private compartment, say so when you make your reservation. You can hoist your luggage onto overhead racks in your compartment, or keep it in the corridor outside. Usually there are porters to help you with the heavy lifting.

It's a good idea to bring your own bottled water, since European railroads don't guarantee the potability of on-board water. You can also buy drinks and snacks on the train platforms.

Your biggest risk in European train travel is getting on the wrong car, thanks to the custom of splitting trains in mid-journey. Your train from Milan to Paris could be split at Dijon, with some cars going to Paris while the rest go south to Lyon. When you board, each car should have a sign on it telling you where it's going.

TRAINS AROUND THE WORLD

There are trains, of course, in every civilized country and some that are not so civilized. You can take a train through Mexico's spectacular Copper Canyon and even stop there overnight, or ride the rails high into the Andes to visit Machu Picchu. You can ride an upholstered car like a rajah through India or speed on a Bullet Train through Japan. You can ride a train great distances through China, across Australia and deep into Africa.

A few countries — like Japan — have their own rail passes. Most countries' railroads outside of Europe do not offer senior discounts. Nevertheless, wherever you plan to travel by train, ask for those discounts.

And remember that riding a train puts you very close to the people and their customs.

RAILROAD DEALS FOR SENIORS

Some national railway systems offer discounts for mature travelers — a saving if you're not traveling on a Eurailpass or a BritRail pass. To get some of the discounts, simply show proof of age at the station when you buy your ticket. For others, you have to buy a low-cost senior-citizens' pass. You can't get these discounts when you buy tickets at home — you have to buy them on the spot. Here are some of them:

Austria — A senior-citizen pass costs $10, gets you half-price on any train for a year. It's for men 65 and over, women 60 and over. You need to have your passport and an extra photo.

Canada — As we noted, Via Rail gives seniors 65 and over one-third off regular fares. Just show proof of age.

Denmark — Those 65 and over get 50 per cent off most days; Friday and Sunday travel is only 25 percent off.

Finland — Those 65 and over get 50 percent off, but you have to travel 48 miles or more.

France — Carte Vermeil for travelers 62 and older costs $20, is good for half-fares on any train for a year during off-peak periods.

Great Britain — Senior Citizen BritRail Passes, good for eight, 15, 22 or 30 days, are 15 percent off regular BritRail Pass rates.

Greece — Those 60 and over get 50 percent off regular fares.

Italy — Women 60 and over and men 65 and over can buy senior-citizen passes for $4 at any railroad station, get 30 percent off regular fares for a year.

Norway — Travelers 67 or older get half off regular fares.

Portugal — Those 60 and over get discounts ranging from 30 percent to 50 percent.

Sweden — Those 65 and over get 30 percent off regular fares.

West Germany — A senior-citizen pass (free) gets those 60 and older half off regular fares.

IN SUMMARY:

— Train travel is often a trip into the nostalgic past.
— Though Amtrak's senior fare is usually no bargain, its All Aboard America pass is one of the best travel buys around.

— For train travel, you need to pack an overnight bag.

— Eurailpasses and BritRail Passes are for tourists planning to visit several cities in a fairly short time.

— If you can't use those passes, most European rail networks have senior-citizen discounts that can save you money.

★ ★ ★
Travel Tool
★ ★ ★

A DOZEN GREAT TRAIN RIDES FOR 49ERS-PLUS

Here are some of the world's best — or at least, most exciting — trains, and how to book them:

Alaska — The Alaska Railroad's Anchorage-Fairbanks run makes breathtaking scenic day-trips in the shadow of Denali (Mt. McKinley). It features 1950s Scenadome cars from Santa Fe's great El Capitan. Get tickets from Alaska State Railroad ☎ (800/544-0582) or Gray Line in Anchorage or Seattle. Gray Line ☎ (toll-free 800/544-2206) and Princess Tours ☎ (toll-free 800/835-8907) operate private cars and tours of Denali State Park on this train.

Canada — The continent's longest rail trip is on Via Rail's Canadian — 3,639 miles in four days from Halifax to Vancouver via Montreal. The best viewing is from Vancouver to Calgary through the Canadian Rockies. TIP: for better viewing, go eastbound. ☎ Call 800/665-0200 for a brochure.

China/Russia — American tourists get two trains for the price of one. After sightseeing in Hong Kong and points in China, travelers board air-conditioned cars of the Trans-Mongolian Express in Beijing bound for Ulan Bator, the Mongolian capital on the edge of the Gobi Desert. Then travelers cross into the Soviet Union, visit Irkutsk and board the fabled Trans-Siberian Express for Moscow. The longest continuous time on the train is four days/three nights. Contact Adventure Center, 5540-TMT College Ave., Oakland, CA 94618, ☎ toll-free 800/227-8747, in California 800/228-8747.

Europe — The "train of kings and the king of trains," the Venice Simplon-Orient-Express is probably the world's most famous train ride. This is the restored grande dame that ruled the rails of Europe during the 1920s. On board, it is once again La Belle Epoque, a world of brass and Lalique crystal and inlaid mahogany, where gentlemen dress for dinner and ladies clutch white gloves. The Orient Express makes the 32-hour trip from London to Venice or Vienna twice a week in season. Despite its name, the Venice leg bypasses the Simplon Tunnel, crossing the northern Alps on the more scenic Arlburg route. The Vienna leg runs east through the towering Kitzbueheler Alps. Passengers can board or stop off at Paris, Innsbruck and Salzburg. Venice Simplon-Orient-Express, One World Trade Center, Ste. 2565, New York, NY 10048, ☎ toll-free 800/524-2420, in Canada 800/451-2253.

India — The weekly Palace on Wheels uses the luxurious old salon cars that carried the maharajas and puka sahibs during the days of the raj. Passengers live aboard in 13 sleeper cars during the seven-day round-trip tour from Delhi through Jaipur, Jodhpur, Agra and other famous points. The train stops frequently for sightseeing tours. Government of India Tourist Office, 30 Rockefeller Plaza, New York, NY 10112 ☎ 212/586-4901.

Mexico — Day trains run the spectacular Copper Canyon route from Chihuahua to Los Mochas in 14 hours. This is a favorite for RV caravaners, who enter Mexico through El Paso and piggyback their rigs on the train. You can stop overnight at lodges in the canyon. Book through one of two tour operators: Romero's Mexican Service, ☎ 714/548-8931, or Turimex, 619/690-2444 in California, toll-free 800/225-6943.

Scotland — The Royal Scotsman, probably Europe's most exclusive train, has trips ranging from 24 hours to seven days. Operating through November from Edinburgh through the Highlands to east and west coasts, it carries only 28 passengers, and has a guide on board. There are gourmet meals on board in a 100-year-old dining car, as well as some at local restaurants. The saloon car is only 75 years old. Abercrombie & Kent, 1420 Kensington Rd., Oak Brook, IL 60521, ☎ toll-free 800/323-7308.

South Africa — Not a vintage train, the famous Blue Train linking Capetown, Johannesburg and Pretoria is widely considered the best modern train in the world. It runs three times a week in high season. SARtravel, Ltd., 370 Lexington Ave., New York, NY 10017, ☎ toll-free 800/727-7207.

Spain — In the north, the Transcantabrico operates over the longest narrow-gauge line in Europe, 625 miles along Spain's rugged north coast between Leon and El Ferrol. Guests sleep aboard the modern train during the seven-day trip, which features side trips to local historic and scenic sites. Breakfast is on board, but most other meals are at local restaurants. National Tourist Office of Spain, 665 Fifth Ave., New York, NY 10022, ☎ 212/759-8822 for a list of wholesalers.

The classic Al Andalus makes three- and four-day trips from Málaga to Seville in southern Spain, with sightseeing stops at Granada and Córdoba. The train carries paneled sleepers, restaurant and bar cars featuring fine inlaid woodwork. Marsans International, 205 E. 42nd St., New York, NY 10017 ☎ toll-free 800/223-6114.

United States — The Coast Starlight from Seattle to Los Angeles, and the California Zephyr from Chicago to San Francisco create a great West Coast trip on the Amtrak. The combined trip under Amtrak's All-Aboard America fares cost $239 and three stopovers are allowed. Information at any Amtrak station or from Amtrak Distribution Center, P.O. Box 7717, Itasca, IL 60143, ☎ toll-free 800/872-7245.

NOTES

CHAPTER 15

FLYING

It's the Quickest — And the Cheapest —
Way To Get There

Flying gives the mature traveler seven-league boots. It is not the most elegant, nor the most comfortable, way to get there — but it is certainly the quickest, and often for seniors, the cheapest.

And that old bogeyman of air travel, fear of flying, has all but disappeared as the number of air passengers soars and the word gets around that, statistically, you're slightly safer in an airplane seat than you are in your bathtub.

Even so, flying can be stressful. To paraphrase an old saw, if God had meant man to fly, He'd have given him 10-foot legs (to make the dash between connecting flights), four arms (to wrestle all the luggage and tickets) and a 10-inch rear end (to fit into six-abreast airline seats).

Nevertheless, planning ahead can take lots of the hassle out of flying, freeing you to have a chuckle at the frequent disputes between airline employees and those passengers who didn't plan ahead.

THE EARLY-BIRD SEATS

Start with seating — perhaps a month before your flight. When you order your ticket, get a seat assignment to go with it — do not put off the seat assignment, as many do, until check-in time. Truly, nobody wants a center seat, and if you put off getting a seat assignment until check-in time, you're almost guaranteed one.

Most passengers choose aisle seats so they can get up and walk around, stretch or go to the john without disturbing seatmates. If you want to sit with someone who also likes an aisle seat, ask for seats across from each other, so you can chat across the aisle.

Window seats are preferred by those who don't like to be disturbed by others getting in an out, and who like to keep track of where the plane is. Besides, the only place you can see the scenery unimpeded is from a window seat. If watching scenery or cloud formations interests you make sure to ask for a window seat that is not over the wings.

If you're troubled by motion sickness, on the other hand, wing seats are the most stable in the airplane — if you sit near the tail, you could get a bucking.

Your other choice in seats on U. S. airlines will be smoking or non-smoking sections if your flight lasts more than two hours. On shorter flights, smoking is forbidden. Some carriers prohibit smoking altogether.

When we fly together, we ask for one seat on the aisle, another by the window. If the center seat isn't sold, there is plenty of room to stretch out. If it is sold, we simply offer to trade one of our more-desirable seats for the center one so we can stay together.

RECONFIRMING YOUR FLIGHT

A day or two before departure — on both ends of your journey — call to reconfirm your flight. Though airlines now try to discourage reconfirming for domestic flights (it takes office workers' time), it can sometimes save your seats.

Airline computers lose return bookings, or they can accidentally wipe out your ticket. The airline might change a flight time and fail to tell you about it. If you wait until you get to the airport, it may be too late to correct any mistake.

When you reconfirm for your return flight, give the airline your room number as well as your hotel's phone number.

GETTING TO THE AIRPORT

A taxi is an expensive way to get to the airport, if you're in most big cities, where airports often are built 20 or 30 miles outside of town. And driving your own car and parking it for the duration can be even more expensive.

Some cities, like Kansas City, have airporter buses on regular schedules from downtown hotels and other pickup points. The cabfare from your home to a pickup point will be fairly cheap. And the cabbie and the bus driver will handle your bags.

Something new in some large cities is the Super Shuttle — usually a large van that picks up or drops off several passengers at once. You call the Super Shuttle number from home, or when you arrive after your flight — it's in the white pages under "Super Shuttle." It picks you up usually within 30 minutes and drops you off at the airport or your hotel. The Super Shuttle driver can schedule a pickup for your return trip on the spot. And they even take credit cards.

Super Shuttle usually costs one-third to half the comparable taxi fare — $12 from Los Angeles International to mid-Wilshire, for example, or $8 into downtown San Francisco. But that is the cost per person, and you still might save a little if you can share a taxi with others. Other Super Shuttle operations are in Phoenix and Dallas-Fort Worth.

The Super Shuttle idea is taking hold rapidly in other cities, and if the Super Shuttle doesn't operate in your town yet, check the phone book for other companies that provide the same type of door-to-door service.

THE BAGGAGE GAME

One good reason to get to the airport early is to beat the jam-up at the baggage check-in. Studies show that a bag arriving at the last minute is more likely to get lost than one that arrives early — no doubt because clerks make more mistakes when they're rushed.

You'll head off back problems if you pack two smaller suitcases instead of a single big one — it will be a balanced load in case you have to carry them across some airport.

But don't try to carry your own bags through the airport if there's a better way. Most airports have curbside check-in — just drop your bags there, get your claim check and head straight to the gate where your flight is leaving.

If you can't find a Skycap to help with your bags, most airports have baggage carts, which look like cut-down grocery carts, for rent. They hold a surprising amount of luggage, and for $1 or its equivalent in foreign currency, you can save a lot of back strain if you have to carry bags across the airport.

As we noted earlier, pack as if you plan to lose your luggage — put irreplaceable items in a carry-on bag, and plan to keep it with you. Here are some other precautions you can take to keep your bags from getting lost:

• Use sturdy bags that won't rip or crack if they're handled roughly. Put a heavy strap around each bag to slow down thieves. And make sure your bags are locked.

• Identify your bags with clearly printed covered tags attached to the handles. One airline executive says you should further identify your bag by tying a ribon around the handle. "We have a lot of gray Sampsonites in the world," he explains.

• Put additional identification inside each bag, along with a copy of your itinerary.

• Remove old destination tags from your bags before check-in.

• After the baggage handler puts the destination tags on your luggage, look to make sure they're for the right destination.

• Once your flight arrives, go right to the baggage-claim area to make sure no one takes your bags and scoots.

Each passenger can check through two bags. In addition, most airlines also limit passengers to two carry-on bags apiece, not counting women's purses. But the size as well as the number of carry-ons can vary, depending on airline policy and the kind of airplane, so check before you make your final packing plans.

Usually passengers are required to check through bulky items like skis and golf bags.

CARRYING PETS

Pets are a special kind of baggage. Each airline has different rules for carrying pets on board. We have seen big dogs tranquilized in portable kennels and put aboard with the baggage. We suppose the dog usually arrives okay — but we wouldn't do that to our dog.

Nevertheless, that's the only way for a pet to travel on some airlines, like Delta and Continental, which do not permit animals — large or small — in the cabin. One airline, Southwest, won't carry pets at all.

Most airlines, on the other hand, will permit small pets to ride with their owners if they'll fit into 7- or 9-inch carriers under the seat. All but TWA require that the pet stay in the kennel during the whole flight. Some airlines have a limit of one pet per flight in the passenger cabin, so you have to reserve the flight as soon as you can to get the "pet slot." Check with the airline well before your trip. Put as much thought into your pet's trip as you do on yours.

There is usually an extra charge for carrying a pet in the luggage compartment, something like $25 to $30 each way.

And find out from the reservation clerk whether a health certificate or proof of shots will be required, and how current they have to be. Piedmont, for instance, wants to see a health certificate issued 10 days earlier or less.

And, of course, you must comply with any animal quarantines at your destination. Great Britain, for example, might quarantine your dog, healthy or not, for up to six months.

LOST BAGGAGE

Yes, the airlines lose people's luggage. On one out of every 30 round trips you make, checking through two bags each time, the odds are you'll lose one bag. And chances are also that the loss will be just temporary.

If your bag is one of the few that winds up missing, report it immediately — before you leave the airport — to a customer-service representative. For a start, the rep can often give you money on the spot for emergency purchases of toilet articles and some clothing. Though the airline hopes to reunite you and your bags within a few hours, it will help you further if there's more delay. It depends, of course, on your persistence and the nature of your trip.

If you're a maestro with a concert to perform that night, the airline no doubt would rent you a tux. It might rent you skis, if yours turn up missing on a ski excursion — but not if you're returning from one. If weeks go by, the airline could wind up buying you a whole new wardrobe. Legally, though, a U. S. airline's liability is limited to $1,250 per passenger. For international travel, the maximum an airline will compensate you is about half that much.

Some airlines offer excess-valuation insurance, which increases that limit — but before you buy it, check your own homeowner's insurance policy to find out what's covered if your luggage goes astray.

If your bag doesn't turn up at all, you must file a written claim, with a list of lost items, when you bought them and how much you paid for them. At this point, the delays could be infuriating. Lost-luggage fraud is rampant, and airline claims departments do everything they can to thwart such claims — including snarling your own claim in red tape. Once you've filed a claim, hang on to a copy of it, your baggage check and your copy of the airline ticket — this is, after all, your only proof you were really on the flight.

If you find the airline has damaged your luggage, report it and insist on completing the airline's damage-report form before you leave the airport. Most airlines will repair or replace any damaged luggage and its contents based on its depreciated value.

GETTING THROUGH THE AIRPORT

In flying, the big congestion is on the ground. Most of our major airports were built before deregulation, which changed the way airlines operate. So plan on plenty of walking.

Domestic airlines nowadays use a hub-and-spoke system, which probably gets passengers where they're going faster and more efficiently. It certainly makes them walk faster through airports. Unless you're taking one of the few cross-country, non-stop flights, you'll start out at the rim, fly down the spoke into the hub, and fly out another spoke to your destination.

If you're taking Delta from San Francisco to Minneapolis, for instance, you'll take one flight into Salt Lake City, and another out to Minneapolis. If you're on American from Miami to Los Angeles, you'll hub through Dallas. All the flights are timed to arrive at about the same time, so they can exchange passengers, and fly out at about the same time. Between 9 and 10 every morning, and at other hub times daily, it looks like every plane Delta owns is on the ground in Salt Lake.

The catch is what you have to do while you're on the ground. These are big airports, and the airlines that hub through them usually have three or four concourses. For reasons we have not yet heard explained, you almost always fly in one end of an airport and fly out of the other — spending your time between flights walking from concourse to concourse.

At Atlanta, where both Delta and Eastern hub, each concourse averages 2,100 feet in length. At Salt Lake City, you walk across three concourses to connect on Delta flights. Making a connecting flight through TWA's hub in St. Louis, a writer for *Conde Nast's Traveler* walked 3,115 feet from gate-to-gate — more than half-a-mile.

If your incoming flight is late, you may have no more than 10 or 15 minutes to make that kind of walk. Often, the airlines will hold flights a few minutes to take care of passengers from a late incoming flight. Sometimes, though, the connecting plane just goes without you.

Fortunately, most of the 34 airports where airlines hub have moving sidewalks for one-third to one-half the distance. You can get on and stand still for a few minutes, or even walk along them as you're moving. If you're in a rush to make connections, though, the moving sidewalks move slower than most people walk, so you're better off on foot.

Even if you're not handicapped, you can get a wheelchair and often an attendant to get you through the airport. In some airports, like Miami, there's a charge for the service. Let the reservation clerk know you need one when you get your ticket, and you'll be met with a wheelchair at every step along the way when boarding or deplaning.

Most airports also have motorized carts, slightly larger than golf carts, that can carry three or four people plus driver from concourse to concourse.

Just ask where to pick up a ride when you check in.

THOSE X-RAY MACHINES

At security checkpoints, you'll be asked to run all your hand-luggage through an X-ray machine. Keep your film away from those things, no matter what the attendant tells you.

Ask the attendant to check camera and film by hand.

X-rays can fog your film, and the more checkpoints you have to go through, the more damage there is — the effects of the X-rays are cumulative on film. Also, the higher the speed of your film, the more likely fogging will occur.

You can ask for hand-checks at any U.S. airport, and at most airports overseas. But in a few more-security-conscious countries that have been targets of terrorism — Italy and France, for example — they will insist that you run your film through the X-rays, no matter how you plead.

Even in the United States, when terminals are crowded the inspector may not have time for a hand-check, or may just take the film from your hand and thrust it into the machine — another good reason for arriving for your flight before the crowd does.

If you're going to request hand-checks, make it easy on the inspector. Have all your film out of its boxes. Though some experts advise putting it in a clear vinyl bag so the inspector can see it, we carry our film in double-lined lead shield bags, which the inspector is free to open. The lead shield protects film if, for some reason, it has to go through the X-rays. We pack our film at the very top of our carry-on bag, so we can get to it easily, and sling our cameras over our shoulders.

If your camera doesn't have a removable lens, as most good 35mm cameras do, don't load film into the camera — for the hand-checker is going to want to peer inside.

Don't pack your film or camera in your suitcases to avoid the check-point X-rays. Though bags are usually not X-rayed, some airports make spot-checks, and the X-ray dosage will be much stronger than that used on hand luggage.

If you know you're going through an airport that won't hand-check your film, a lead-shield bag is the only way to pack it. You can buy the bags, which carry up to 20 rolls, at any camera store. Inside these bags, your film probably will be safe, especially if it's a slow-speed film. Any film under 1000 ASA can usually take one dose of X-ray without harm. Slower film, like Kodak's

24 ASA and 64 ASA Kodachrome slide films, can stand several X-ray passes before there's visible fogging, according to the manufacturer.

There's still a debate on whether the X-ray machines are harmful to portable computers. One manufacturer, TRS Radio Shack, warns that "X-ray machines have been known to wipe out the memory in the Model 100. X-ray machines operating in the vicinity of any computer can cause damage to that unit." That could include pocket calculators or any electronic games you plan to play aboard the plane. Have those hand-checked, too, if you can.

As far as anyone knows, there seem to be no harmful effects from X-rays on video recorders or their tapes, so those can go through the machines safely.

IF YOU GET BUMPED

Airlines are permitted to do a certain amount of overbooking — selling more seats than there are on the plane. After all, there are always a few who don't show up and haven't canceled, and without overbooking, a plane could fly with lots of empty seats.

The other side of that coin is that, occasionally, there'll be more passengers with confirmed reservations than there are seats for them. The result is that some passengers get "bumped" — held over for a future flight.

Usually you have a 1-in-3,000 chance of getting bumped — even less if you fly midweek. But the odds more than double in December, with everyone going somewhere for the holidays.

When a plane is oversold, the first thing the airline does is ask for volunteers to give up their seats in return for cash or a free ticket. Before you volunteer, figure out whether getting bumped will cost you more than whatever the airline is offering. Will the airline pay for your meals while you're stranded? Or your hotel bill? What would a delay do to your travel plans on the other end? Would you miss Susie's graduation, or the sailing of your cruiseship?

If there are not enough volunteers to get off the plane, the next step is involuntary bumping. And most airlines select those to be bumped on a last-at-the-gate, first-bumped basis — another good reason for getting to the airport early for check in.

If the airline can place you on another flight that is scheduled to arrive within an hour of your original flight, you won't receive any compensation. If the airline puts you on a flight arriving between one and two hours later than your original flight, you'll get an amount equal to the fare on your oversold flight (up to $200). And if they can't get you there within two hours of the original arrival time, you'll get twice the fare of your oversold flight, up to $400. The airline has to give you a check or free tickets right away.

Sometimes your flight is canceled or delayed for hours, and if it's the airline's fault, your big gun is Rule 240. The airline has to book you on a competing airline at no additional cost. The trick is getting through to the airline's passenger agent, when 200 others on the plane are trying to do the same thing. Instead, go to a telephone and make reservations on the competing airline. Then, when you finally get to the passenger agent, you've already got a confirmed seat. Say simply, "I want to invoke Rule 240," and ask the agent to endorse your ticket.

AIRPORT TAXES

A hidden zinger for international travelers is the airport tax — in effect, a charge for letting you out of the country.

Supposedly, the per-capita tax is to pay for airport maintenance, and you simply can't leave the country until you pay it. The tax can range from $1 or so in Auckland to more than $15 (US) in Hong Kong.

Often you're not told about the tax until you get to the airport — after you've packed your bags and gotten rid of all your foreign currency. For that reason, many airports let you pay the tax in U.S. dollars.

AIRLINES' DEALS FOR SENIORS

Almost all domestic airlines now have discount programs for mature travelers. They feel that we represent a choice group of customers who can help fill empty seats. The airlines want us because we have an inclination to visit relatives more often, have more flexibility in travel schedules than most people and are overcoming previous fears of flying.

Airlines for years have been successful in wooing business travelers. But that strategy has resulted in relatively empty airplanes at midweek and on Saturdays, airline marketing executives tell us. The airlines have figured out that seniors, if given discounts, are the most likely group to fill these seats.

Typical restrictions on the senior-discount programs reflect this empty-seat strategy:

• You can fly only on Tuesdays, Wednesdays, Thursdays and Saturdays in most programs.

• You can't purchase tickets earlier than six days before your first leg (you can buy return tickets at the same time).

• On some airlines, the number of seats is limited.

But for most seniors, the restrictions are worth it: typical discounts are 10 to 15 percent below airlines' lowest promotional fares, and much higher discounts are available on selected flights — we've seen fares for seniors discounted up to 50 percent on some America West flights, for example. Though some airline clubs permit those over 60 to join, the real bonanzas start coming to those 62 to 65 or older.

Here is the downside: many senior discounts apply only to regular coach fares. Some airlines offer everyone restricted promotional fares which are even lower than the unrestricted senior fares — an example is Continental, which charges a regular coach fare of $690 round-trip from Kansas City to Reno, Nev. The comparable fare for seniors is $432, but there is a non-refundable promotional fare of $211, which anybody can get just by buying tickets in advance.

If you feel looking for senior discounts gets you right back into the mess of having to shop for fares, you're right. But let your travel agent do the shopping — senior-discount tickets are commissionable to agents, and you might as well let them earn their keep.

To take best advantage of senior-discount programs, try to guess at your travel plans at least a year in advance. Figure out where you're likely to be going, and how often. If an airline that serves your community doesn't fly where you're going, you won't want to join that program.

Read the fine print before you choose an airline deal for seniors. As we said, some airlines won't apply senior discounts to their promotional rates, which in some cases are even steeply lower. And don't be lured by additional discounts at hotels and rent-a-cars — you can get those in a lot of different ways. To use some of these airline deals, you have to join a club and sometimes pay dues; for others, you just have to declare your age.

There are basically three kinds of programs for seniors, plus some variations:

Club deals — These charge a small membership fee, and offer packages of discounts on tours, hotels and rental cars. Usually you can join when you're 60 to get these benefits, but it's not until you turn 65 that you begin getting 10 percent off airline tickets. Continental, Northwest, Piedmont, American, United, TWA and Eastern have clubs. These benefit seniors who travel frequently for pleasure. You enroll in the clubs at airline ticket counters, then book through either travel agents or the airlines. Most of the clubs have arrangements with foreign airlines to extend their discounts for overseas travel.

Coupon books — Seniors 62 and older can buy four- and eight-coupon books good for one-way travel between any two city pairs on the route. Using these coupons, you could fly New York-Los Angeles and back — or between any other cities — for as little as $154. Flying to Honolulu would cost $368 — one of the best fares available outside of a tour package. Piedmont, Delta and Eastern offer coupons. Coupons benefit seniors who make longer hauls, and know where they're going to be going. Buy coupon books either from the airlines or your travel agent.

Senior Passports — Eastern, Continental and TWA offer system-wide passes, good for a year — but some restrictions may be prohibitive. On Eastern, you can fly only three times between city pairs, for example, and Sunday stayovers are required. If you're planning a number of trips where these airlines go, and you plan your travel carefully, these passes can be the best deals of all. If you could use all the flights, Continental's Senior Passport, for example, would permit you to fly anywhere in the United States for less than $62 a round trip.

Straight discounts — You don't have to join anything, and tickets aren't restricted. Just prove your age and step aboard. You get the best promotional rate for the flight you want, then take an additional seniors' discount ranging from 10 to 50 percent. Straight discounts benefit seniors who make shorter flights, and can't plan their travel months ahead. Either the airline or a travel agent can book these tickets. Among airlines with straight discounts are Braniff, Continental, American West and Delta.

And don't forget that discount travel agencies (see Chapter 3, Your Friend The Travel Agent) can save you additional dollars, once you've decided to take part in a particular program — especially one of the high-priced ones. Delta's four-coupon deal, regularly priced at $368, costs seniors only $347 at McTravel Travel Services in Chicago. You can buy Eastern's $1,299 Get Up And Go Passport at McTravel for $1,203.

A list of current airline deals for seniors follows this chapter.

Airlines sometimes stage short-term promotions for seniors, in addition to their regular deals. Eastern and Continental in the past have cut summer rates for seniors; America West posts low senior citizen fares for particular destinations.

Just like you do when making lodging reservations, always ask the airline ticket clerk whether there's a senior citizen rate — even if you're under 65.

IN SUMMARY

— Flying is the quickest way to get there — but not the most comfortable.

— Make your flight arrangements early — and get to the airport early.

— You have a 30-1 chance against losing a bag — but the airlines will help you when you do.

— Plan on plenty of walking through airports, but there is a way to ride.

— Keep your film away from those airport X-rays.

— If you get bumped from your flight, make sure you get even.

— Almost every airline has deals or discounts for seniors. Ask for them.

★ ★ ★
Travel Tool
★ ★ ★

AIRLINE DEALS FOR 49ERS-PLUS

This listing is compiled from *The Mature Traveler* newsletter's annual survey of airline deals for 49ers-plus. Airlines can change the terms of any offer on short notice:

Air Canada — Has complicated fare discounts for those 65 and older that seem to range up to 50%, depending on city pairs. Most require 14-day advance purchase, with Saturday-night stopovers. Flies from eastern U.S. cities into Canada, and across the continent. ☎ Phone for details and quotes, 800/422-6232.

Alaska Airlines — Travelers 60 and over get deep discounts on some fares in and out of Alaska — the percentage varies according to destination. ☎ Call 800/426-0333.

Aloha Airlines — Non-resident seniors over 65 fly anywhere in the Hawaiian Islands for $37.95 one-way, a 15.6% saving over regular fare of $44.95. ☎ 800/367-5250.

American Airlines — Senior SAAvers club for those over 60 costs $25 (lifetime), offers discounts on tours and hotels. At 65, members get 10% off all American and American Eagle fares without restriction. Companion membership (for those under 65, when you're flying together) is $100. American flies to most U.S. cities, plus Canada, Europe and the Caribbean. ☎ To enroll, call 800/433-7300.

American West — Offers variable "Preferred Senior" fares everywhere it's not in competition with Eastern or Continental, and matches the other airlines' senior deals in those places. Also offers passengers 65 or more up to half off on some flights — you have to travel midweek or Saturdays and fly overnight. But you can fly from Chicago to Las Vegas for only $65, for example. ☎ 800/247-5692 to find out about seniors' deals.

Braniff — Any traveler 65 or more is eligible for a 15% discount off almost any fare, and a companion of any age gets the same discount. Braniff, with hubs in Kansas City and Dallas, flies throughout the Midwest and some western points. ☎ 800/272-6433

Continental Airlines — Offers special seniors' fares to those over 65, in addition to Golden Travelers Club for those over 60 and a Senior Passport for those 62 or more. Lifetime club membership is $25, companion option an extra $100. Members get tour, hotel and car rental discounts, 10% off airfares for members 65 or more. Passport, costing $1,299, is good for 42 legs each year in the U.S. mainland — less than $62 a round trip, if you use them all. Continental flies to most major U.S. cities as well as overseas. ☎ 800/525-6280.

Delta Air Lines — "Young At Heart" coupons for those 62 or more cost $384 for four, $640 for eight, are each good for one leg of travel anywhere on Delta's system for one year — a round trip takes two coupons; Hawaii and Alaska take four coupons. Restrictions: travel is limited to midweek and Saturdays; you book seats six days or less in advance; and they're limited on most flights. Basically, you go when the airline wants you to go, but coupon prices represent substantial savings. Delta flies nationwide and to Mexico and the Caribbean. Buy Young At Heart coupons at any travel agency or Delta ticket office. ☎ 800/221-1212.

Eastern Air Lines — Has three deals for seniors. Senior Citizens Card (a club deal) costs $25, has same age limits, benefits as American's. Seniors' coupons, at $368 (four) and $618 (eight), have same restrictions as Delta's, except travel can start at noon Mondays. Get-Up-And-Go-Passport, at $1,299, offers passengers 62 or more one flight a week anywhere on the domestic system for a year. Travel is limited to midweeks and Saturdays; one leg a week; no more than three trips to any one city; seven days or less advance booking; Sunday layover required; no travel on blackout dates. Companion Passport costs the same; Caribbean Passport costs $1,499; and a First Class Passport is $1,799. "Money's Worth Refund Policy" guarantees savings. For club application, ☎ 800/327-8376. Eastern flies nationwide. Buy coupons and Passports at any travel agency or Eastern ticket office.

Hawaiian Air — Passengers 65 or more fly any inter-island hop for $37.95, 15.6% off the regular fare of $44.95. ☎ 800/367-5320.

Mexicana — Gives 10% discounts on all fares to passengers 65 or more. Flies from U.S. gateways into Mexico. ☎ 800/531-7921.

Midwest Express — Those 65 or older get 10% off all quoted fares. Midwest flies east and south out of Milwaukee. ☎ 800/452-2022.

Northwest Airlines — WorldHorizons Club costs $50 for lifetime membership, gives travelers 65 or more 10% off on all fares, plus range of discounts on hotels, rental cars, special trips. When you join, you get two $25 flight credits — free money. Northwest flies to most major U.S. cities, Canada, Mexico and Jamaica, and a few points in Europe and Asia. Write World-Horizons, P.O. Box 1735, Minneapolis, MN 55440, or call ☎ 800/777-8585.

Pan American — Mid-day and weekend shuttle flights from New York to Boston or Washington cost travelers 65 or more only $45, compared with regular fares of $69-$89. You have to fly between 10:30 a.m.-2:30 p.m or 7:30-9:30 p.m. weekdays, all day Saturdays or until 8:30 p.m. Sundays. ☎ 800/221-1111.

Southwest Airlines — Offers special fares to travelers over 64 that vary from city to city, with none over $99 one way. Fly all over Texas for $19 a leg, for example — also from Detroit to Chicago. Southwest flies mostly in the southwestern U.S., including Texas. Phone local numbers.

TWA — Has two deals. Senior Travel Pass, similar to Eastern's, is $1,399. Senior Travel Club is similar to American's. TWA is a nationwide carrier, with international routes, as well. To join, ☎ phone 800/221-2000. Buy travel passes through travel agents or TWA ticket counters.

United Air Lines — Silver Wings Plus Travel Club costs $50, but whole thing is credited to the first ticket purchased. Also offers 10% discounts on KLM, Lufthansa, Alitalia and British Airways to those 65 or more. Other details are similar to American's. United flies nationwide. To join, ☎ call 800/628-2868.

USAir — Gives 10 percent off all fares to those over 65, and a companion of any age flies at the same price. USAir is a nationwide airline. ☎ 800/428-4322.

III

BEING THERE

Now that you've arrived at your destination, here's
how to get the most out of it.

CHAPTER 16

GETTING YOUR BEARINGS

> Your Visit Doesn't Start Until You Can Find
> Your Way Around

Our first time in San Francisco we never got to Chinatown, didn't visit the waterfront, didn't ride a cable car, were within a block of North Beach and couldn't find Telegraph Hill. It was the time of the "little winter" — a typical miserable, misty July day with the fog so thick we couldn't see more than three blocks down Market Street. And we had only one day to tour.

We were youngsters then — without a city map, without a guidebook, without a guide, wondering what we were supposed to be seeing in the magical city by the bay. We ended up watching a foreign movie on Market Street and, later, having a drink at the soon-to-be-legendary hungry i nightclub — highlights of the visit. Magical San Francisco, huh?

Some years later, we returned, spent the first full day on a guided limousine tour with eight other people, learned you can find your way to any place in San Francisco if you keep Coit Tower in sight, heard a lot of inside stories about a lot of inside places from our knowledgeable guide. Of course, once we could find our way around, we lost our hearts . . .

And so it goes in any strange new city. Your visit doesn't begin until you can find your way around.

THE CITY TOUR

Whenever we visit a new city now, we take a city tour — we look for a tour lasting at least a half-day in small cities, a full day in big ones. We think the city tour is vital if you're going to get your bearings and enjoy a city. We don't waste any time — we take it the first full day there.

Without knowing anything else about the tour company, we check the hotel racks for a Grey Line tour folder. Grey Line is not a company; rather, it's an international association of nearly 175 local tour companies that band together for marketing. They know that if your Grey Line tour of San Francisco is good this year, you'll take the Grey Line tour of Amsterdam next year.

If we can't find a Grey Line tour, we'll look for another reputable company we've heard of, like Thomas Cook or American Express. After that, we ask the concierge to recommend a tour. And we also ask the concierge, "Have you been on the tour? Where does it go? Is it a complete look at the area? Is the tour commentary given in English?"

You can never ask too many questions. On our first trip through London, we took what was called "The City" tour, and wondered why it only lasted a half-day in such a big place. Of course, we found out that "The City" is only that mile-square historic district that includes the Tower of London, and Tower Bridge, St. Paul's and a few other landmarks — but not the Parliament, Westminster Abbey, Kensington Palace, Piccadilly Circus, the shopping district, the West End theater district and a host of London's other famous sites. Those were on a separate London tour — and during our short stay (we were on the way to somewhere else), we had to put that tour off till later.

In many cities, you can arrange for the tour before you leave home by asking your travel agent to book the most complete city tour available.

SPOTTING THE LANDMARKS

When you're on the city tour, bring along a map and make notes.

You have to know how to locate places you want to return to from your hotel, unless you want to get lost or be at the mercy of taxi drivers.

A sightseeing tour is not all "seeing," either. You have purchased the time of a knowledgeable native. Ask the tour guide whatever you need to know — what are the best restaurants, the best museums, the best shopping places, the most dangerous areas of town. What are local customs you need to know to get along with the natives?

Use the tour to get a line on major landmarks. If you know that the Seine runs east-west through Paris, and that Notre Dame is on an island in the middle of it, and that your hotel is upstream (or downstream) from it, you can always find Notre Dame — and your hotel.

You can get your bearings easily in cities with prominent landmarks. If you kept your eye on Coit Tower, the highest point in town, it was impossible to be lost in San Francisco. If you remember that Georgetown is northwest of the Washington Monument, or north across the river from the Lee Mansion in Arlington, you can always find Georgetown because you can see the Lee Mansion and the monument from almost anyplace in town.

Big, flat cities like London and Paris are more trouble navigating. Your best bet in most cities is to remember where the river is, or the ocean-front, and go in a particular direction from there. Even that doesn't always work in towns like San Diego, where the bay can be on three sides of you. In earlier days we always knew where we were in San Diego by the direction of the brightly lighted El Cortez Hotel, high on a hill overlooking downtown.

Towns with tangled streets that never seem to go straight to where you want are also difficult — all the old European cities are that way. In those, the best you can do is keep in mind where three or four major thoroughfares go, and get your bearings from those. And as for using canals, like those in Amsterdam or Venice, as landmarks, forget it — you've seen one canal, you've seen 'em all. But any city laid out on grids, like New York or Chicago, will be fairly easy, because you can navigate by the street numbers.

And, alas, just when you think you know a city well enough to get around in it, things change. San Diego's El Cortez is hidden behind a wall of skyscrapers nowadays, and from inside San Francisco's new highrise canyons, you can't even see Coit Tower. For the first time since we were kids, we're getting lost in the magic city.

CARE AND FEEDING OF TOUR GUIDES

Many tour guides are professionals — not just chamber of commerce types who are proud to have you see their city. In England there are guilds (unions) of tour guides that enforce rigorous standards and have tough training periods.

"It's not just the history of this place, or who is buried where that we are tested on," a guide at St. Paul's Cathedral told us. "We have to know the location of the loos (restrooms), the closest emergency medical center and the bus schedules outside the door."

In the United States, there are schools for tour guides, just like business and beauty schools.

When you sign up for a tour, try to get one with a guide who speaks English — or at least one with a multilingual presentation that includes English. You don't want to spend half-a-day on a bus hearing a guide explain the complicated culture or seeing things you can't possibly understand.

Overseas, you're expected to tip the guide and driver at the end of your tour (see Chapter 19, Tipping). Remember, the guide usually splits tips with the bus driver. A dollar per person is enough for a short tour, $2 to $5 for a longer tour. Though it's not the custom, we think it's nice to tip guides in America, too. After all, they work just as hard as their foreign counterparts. And, because it's not expected, it's ever-so-much more appreciated.

OVERCOMING LANGUAGE BARRIERS

You can travel anywhere in the world and get by with nothing but English. But it's a lot more fun if you know some of the local language.

We were in a hotel elevator in Acapulco, about to turn in for the night, when some of the mariachi bandsmen stepped aboard, chattering away. We don't speak Spanish, but we knew from the tone of their voices and their sly smiles that they were making great fun of us *gringos*.

As the elevator got underway, one of them asked in broken English what floor we wanted.

"*Ocho*," said the sly lady traveler — probably the only word of Spanish she knew.

And the musicians' chatter stopped instantly. Her accent must have been pretty convincing. They were very polite to us as we left the elevator on "ocho" (the eighth floor).

Since then, we have flirted in broken German ("*Wie gehts, Liebchen*"), gotten a car fixed with our broken French ("*L'auto — il fait pooooof!*"), played blackjack with our broken Italian ("busted, *grat-zee*") and wandered around any number of other countries pointing, smiling, nodding and generally communicating pretty well with just a few local phrases.

What we have learned is that in most countries, the people appreciate it when you try to use their language. Your mistakes are jolly good fun, and everyone is pleased that you are willing to try. Your triumphs are their triumphs, and everyone is proud of you. Whether bargaining over a trinket, asking for directions or complimenting someone for a job well done, a big smile, some body English and a small dose of native phrases will go a long way toward making friends.

We emphasize that a small dose is all you need. If you've had high-school French or Spanish, that may be enough. If you live in a big city, chances are there will be an Italian club, a German club or whatever that sponsors short courses in their language for tourists. It's easier, of course, to brush up on whatever language skills you had than to start from scratch.

If you're going with a group of people from where you live, hire a language instructor a few weeks before your trip for a quick conversational course. You don't need to learn the whole structure of the language — just a few words. "Restroom?" with a shrug of the shoulders is just as good a question as "Where is the restroom?"

You don't need to be able to tell a Parisian taxi driver, "Please turn up the air conditioning in your cab." All you need is *chaud* — the word for "hot." Just use it and point to the control on his dashboard; he'll get the idea.

If you can't take a brush-up class, another good way to learn a few foreign phrases is to get a Berlitz Travel Kit — they're $14.95 at most bookstores. The kits are mostly cassettes, taped briefings on what to see, what to pack, on museums and foods and restaurants and even some offbeat things to see and do. And, of course, the cassettes give you important words and phrases for the country you're visiting. Berlitz kits are available for France,

Germany, Great Britain, Italy, Mexico, Spain and Switzerland. The kits also come with a pocket-size *Berlitz Travel Guide* containing maps and basic information. If you can't find them in your bookstore, write Macmillan Publishing Co., 800 Third Ave, New York, NY 10022.

You can also buy a foreign dictionary to take along — they're nice to point to when you're in a pickle abroad, but they don't give you the pronunciation like tapes do.

USING THE CONCIERGE

Whenever you find one, let your hotel's concierge take on the research and the routine "work" of travel for you.

Whether they're called "concierges," "hosts" or "hospitality reps," the job of these folks is to make your life easier, your hotel stay a pleasure and your city visit a wonderful adventure.

It was hard to believe, but there was no professional theater anywhere around London — not even at Stratford — staging a Shakespeare play. It seemed to us unthinkable to visit London and not see any Shakespeare. So we laid our problem on the concierge at our hotel.

She spent most of the afternoon phoning around, finally came up with a semi-pro repertory troupe that was doing *Romeo and Juliet* that night in a church many miles away in northeast London. The concierge showed us how to catch the underground, transfer to a bus and walk another half-mile to find the church. The performance was wonderful — better than any professional company we'd seen in the United States.

And when we returned, the concierge's helper asked us how it was and duly made notes to pass on to the next Shakespeare fans who asked.

Truly, the concierge was our friend in a strange new place, our problem solver.

In America, the concierge idea is fairly new. Here, there are only a handful of members of the prestigious Les Clefs d'Or, the international organization of concierges. Most of them are clustered in New York, San Francisco and other entertainment centers. At many American hotels that do not have concierges, the same job is done at hospitality desks or by designated hosts.

Among the routine chores you can ask the concierge/host to do for you:

- Make reservations for theaters, restaurants, night clubs, sports events and the like.
- Arrange car rentals, limousines, drivers, airport vans, tour guides.
- Get you airline tickets, take care of flight changes, reconfirm your reservations.
- Give directions to any place in town, and offer advice on shopping, tipping and local customs.

A good concierge will get you into restaurants when they're booked solid, find you a rental car when there are seemingly none available, tell you what shop will have that just-right gift at the best price (and maybe even go buy it for you).

And if you'll want something really special, you can even phone the concierge in advance of your visit.

Travel & Leisure magazine tells the story of San Francisco's Holly Stiel, concierge for the Hyatt Union Square, who answered the call of a distraught husband begging her to plan a second honeymoon to save his rocky marriage. "I found them a convertible, arranged a picnic lunch and reserved seats at a romantic restaurant and nightclub on Nob Hill where they could dance," said Steil, who was credited with saving the marriage.

In America, most concierges and hosts are employed by the hotel, work for salaries and don't expect tips — though some kind of "thank-you" gesture is always in order. In Europe, however, they're almost all independent contractors, earning their commissions from the lobby personnel — bellhops, doormen and the like — who work at the concierge's pleasure. There seems to be no standard for rewarding a concierge for services rendered — and that's one area in which a discreet concierge won't advise you, either. Some travelers tip a dollar or two for each service rendered; others wait until the end of their stay and leave $25 to $50 in an envelope as they depart. One rule of thumb is to gauge the size of the tip to the services performed — if you have made some unusual request that took the concierge the best part of a day to fulfill, your tip should be larger.

GETTING AROUND TOWN

Taxi drivers, as much as concierges, often have the best inside information, and they, too, work for tips. So all you have to do is ask. Start with the first cabbie who picks you up at the airport; pump him for all the information you can. And keep pumping cabbies your whole visit.

You may have trouble with that overseas, however, where you and the cabbie don't speak the same language. In that event, before you leave for your destination, have the concierge, the desk clerk or your tour guide write down the address of the place you're going in the native language, and show the piece of paper to the driver. If your hotel has a bellman or doorman who speaks English, ask him to instruct the cab driver where to take you.

In this country or abroad, always ask what it's going to cost. In some countries, taxis operate without meters, and the fare is open to bargaining. If you have a choice, don't use a taxi that doesn't have a meter.

Instead of a taxi, it satisfies our sense of adventure to try the mass transit wherever we go — the double-decker buses in London, the trolley in Munich, the sleek BART underground in San Francisco. And it's truly hard to get lost most of the time — you simply cross the street or the tube and get back on the same car going the other way. Besides, we've never seen a subway — whether the people-mover at the Dallas airport or the tangled underground in London — that didn't have exactly the same kind of understandable diagram of stops and stations that you find on the IRT, the El or the Metro.

THE LOCAL CUSTOMS

When in Rome, they say, do as the Romans do. Even if they don't say how you're supposed to know how the Romans do it.

You will make more friends, learn more about a country, have a better trip if you try to blend in. Find out from the guidebooks, magazine articles and other reading as much as you can about the local customs before you get there. Here are some books to start on:

Do's and Taboos Around the World: A Guide to International Behavior by Roger E. Axtell (Wiley Books, New York, 1986; $9.95).

The Travelers' Guide to European Customs and Manners by Nancy L. Braganti and Elizabeth Devine (Meadowbrook Press, Deephaven, Minn., 1984; $6.95).

Survival Kit for Overseas Living by L. Robert Kohls (Intercultural Press, Inc., Yarmouth, Maine, 1984; $6.95).

Living Overseas: A Book of Preparations by Ted Ward (The Free Press, New York, 1985; $9.95).

IN SUMMARY:

— Always start your visit with a guided city tour.
— Spot landmarks to help you find your way.
— Pick up a few local phrases.
— Use the concierge to take the work out of travel.
— Pump the taxi drivers for information.
— Use the mass transit to satisfy your sense of adventure.

CHAPTER 17

SHOPPING

> ## It's the Traveler's No. 1 Pastime

If there's one thing the lady traveler loves to do — no matter where we go — it's to shop.

And if the truth were known, she's not alone. Shopping is the No. 1 recreational activity, not only for travelers, but also for people who stay at home. So popular a pastime is shopping that AAA is about to incorporate information about shopping locations and specialties into its famous tour books.

If that isn't enough proof, consider the number of shopping excursions offered regularly by travel packagers, airlines and hotels. The closer you get to the Christmas season, the more likely you are to find special travel-shopping packages offered by hotels in large cities such as San Francisco or New York. These tours are often advertised or listed in the travel sections of nearby out-of-town newspapers.

SHOP-TILL-YOU-DROP TOURS

Even if Christmas isn't just around the corner, there are special shopping excursions offered to travelers year-round. A recent one was a seven-day shopping tour of Paris for $1,159, including round-trip airfare, accommodations, sightseeing, fashion shows and shopping discounts.

And if you need of a quick shopping fix, there are a number of agencies like CIE Tours International (122 E. 42nd St., New York, NY 10168, ☎ 212/972-5600), which often offers weekend shopping sprees to Ireland, where you can stock up on woolens, crystal, china and more.

If you want to shop in a specific country, give the tourist office or national airline a call. Finnair and Icelandair, for example, sometimes offer shopping weekends at very attractive rates. So, too, do the Milford Plaza in New York and Ritz-Carlton hotels in Atlanta, Boston and Rancho Mirage, Calif.

In some markets, people who know their shops conduct excursions for visitors. Julie Steel (P.O. Box 3262, Auckland (09) 397-442, New Zealand) offers fashion tours of Auckland factory outlets, while in Hawaii, you can contact Hidden Treasures Shopping Excursions (201 Poipu Dr., Honolulu, HI 96825, ☎ 808/395-1756) for shopping outside of the tourist areas.

If you're hunting for such an excursion, ask your travel agent for advice.

You may have noted that the word "buying" hasn't come into play, yet. We're talking shopping, not necessarily buying. Veteran shoppers know that you really don't have to buy anything to enjoy shopping.

For one thing, shopping provides you with insights on the peoples, customs, economies and priorities of the places you visit. At the markets, you'll enjoy a slice of local life — whether it's at the Marche' aux Puces near Paris or Rodeo Drive in Los Angeles, from New York's Fifth Avenue to the tailor shops of Hong Kong, from Harrod's to Neiman-Marcus.

SHOPPING FOR VALUE

The first rule of a good shopper is to know what you're looking for and what's available. If you know that, you're more likely to locate real finds. You wouldn't be wise, for example, to shop for turquoise in Paris. You'd pay import fees as well as local taxes and duty, and a huge overhead. But if you choose a place like New Mexico to hunt for turquoise, you'd find jewelry made of local materials and created by native artists.

Part of our trip preparation is to learn which items are grown or made locally, information often available from the tourist information office. This research serves a second purpose. It helps us to shop for items that are duty-free and to make sure we don't buy items not allowed into the United States.

Our government has a program called the U.S. Generalized System of Preference (GSP), which is an effort to promote the local industries and economies. Between now and July 1993, GSP gives duty-free status to 140 nations, and assures duty-free shopping, provided you buy items that originate in the countries where you make your purchases. In other words, if you buy in Mexico the leather goods made by Mexican artisans or, in India, the wood carvings made by Indian craftsmen, you can exceed the $400 limit and be exempt from paying duty on those items.

To get your free copy of *GSP and the Traveler*, outlining the countries and items included in GSP, write the U.S. Customs Service, Room 201, 6 World Trade Center, New York, NY 10048.

Don't even try to bring home prohibited and restricted items, which range from plants and plant products to Cuban cigars. Write the Customs Service for the free brochure, *Know Before You Go*, publication 512, to make sure that what you want to buy won't be confiscated at customs. The booklet also outlines customs exemptions for U.S. insular possessions like Guam (up to $800 per person) or other countries (up to $400 per person) and describes amounts of duty charged on various imported items and methods of payment.

Here is other research you should do if you're planning a lot of shopping abroad:

• Ask the foreign tourist offices for information on getting Value Added Tax (VAT) refunds.

• Find out what the items you're interested in buying cost in America. That gives you a benchmark to know when you've uncovered a real bargain overseas.

• If you're going to shop for large items such as furniture, find out what packing, insurance, shipping and import duty will add to the cost. Contact a U.S. import firm and ask for advice on reliable shippers in the countries you're visiting.

There are also companies that specialize in shipping heavy goods to the U.S. from overseas. An example is Michael Davis, a London firm which has offices in many different countries. Not only does Michael Davis pick up items from different shops in the same country and consolidate them into a single shipment for packing, it often has advice on the least expensive method of shipment such as standby service, which can save money for large items that have relatively small value. If you find yourself making a large purchase without having done the advance research, the concierge often has good ideas for safe shipment.

• Finally, we familiarize ourselves with the local numbers we'll be dealing with such as the exchange rate (Chapter 6, Money Matters), the currency of the country, and the sizes used for clothing and shoes — a table is at the end of this chapter.

SHOPPING WITH A PURPOSE

We almost always have a list of gifts to be purchased when we travel: birthday items for godchildren, Christmas gifts for relatives, souvenirs for us. If the items to be purchased include clothing, we take along a list of the sizes for the person. That means we have specific things to shop for in each area visited.

Even with such a list, we put other limits on our shopping:

• Not only do we know the best items to shop for in each country, we also try to locate the best local shopping areas and specialty stores. That way we can avoid cookie-cutter shopping malls and canned group places to visit during sightseeing expeditions. Guidebooks tell us some Murano shops in Venice carry glass from all over Italy, maybe even from Korea. So we hold off our glass shopping until we actually visit the nearby island of Murano, where only the local product is sold. We don't shop for lace in Venice, either, until we take a boat to the island of Burano.

• We look for items that are easily carried and comparatively unbreakable, if we plan to carry them home ourselves. That means the antique maps we like to collect should not be framed when we buy them; without frames, they'll fit into a mailing tube, and that mailing tube can fit inside a garment bag or be mailed.

• Whenever we can, we try to buy items valued at $50 or less. That means we can mail them duty- and tax-free. You can mail only one package a day, and you must mark it: "Unsolicited gift, value less than $50" ($40 for Canada) with a description on the outside. If the items are mailed from the store where they're purchased, we also avoid the Value Added Tax (VAT). We always pack mailing labels addressed to people we plan to send gifts to.

THAT VALUE-ADDED TAX

For everything you buy that you plan to carry home with you, get receipts. The receipts serve two purposes. First, they meet the paperwork needs of customs. Second, they can help save money when you apply for a VAT refund.

A VAT is levied in varying amounts on goods sold in Western Europe, Japan and Israel. To be eligible, of course, you have to shop at stores offering VAT refunds. Some announce this with signs saying "Tax Free," while some countries have adopted specific symbols. In England it's a red, white and blue symbol; in Israel it's two figures carrying a cluster of grapes;

After you make the minimum qualifying purchase, ask for a VAT refund form and prove you're a foreign visitor by displaying your passport. The clerk will complete the form and you will sign it.

Stop at customs before leaving the country to file for your refund and to show your purchases. To make this as easy as possible, pack all VAT refund items together so they can be displayed easily.

DOING DUTY-FREE?

Duty-free shops are better described as tax-free shops, because what they are doing is holding goods without paying local taxes on them. You buy items, in effect, before they are admitted to the country in question. But the items purchased at a duty-free shop must be declared when you re-enter the United States. And if the items push you over the $400 exemption or quantity of allowed liquor, you will pay duty on them.

Because of this, those touted bargains are hard to find at some duty-free shops. The shops do serve a function if you need a last-minute gift for someone on your list, if you want to buy liquor to serve in the country you're visiting, or if you know the value of the items you're shopping for. For example, if you know what a specific camera or watch costs at home, and the duty-free shop is offering it to you with a 50 percent discount, you know it's a great deal — grab it!

CUSTOMS CLAIMS

So you won't be charged import duty on your personal belongings, register all foreign-made items — cameras, watches, clothing and the like — with U.S. customs before you leave, and carry the registration certificates with you (see Chapter 7, Your Papers, Please).

When you return, have receipts and items to be declared together and accessible.

If you've bought an antique, have the receipt indicate the age of the item; antiques and art works are admitted duty free.

And be sure to tell the customs agent the truth.

BARGAINING

One person's shopping dream trip is another's confused mess. But if you haven't tried bargaining for an item, you should — it's really part of learning how the rest of the world lives.

Bargaining is not likely to be an operation greeted with open arms at department stores, no matter where you go. But it can be an afternoon's entertainment in street markets throughout the world.

Bargaining is not something that's easy for most American shoppers. We're accustomed to seeing a price tag and paying what it says.

If you want to try your hand at bargaining, here are some tips to help make it easier for you:

• Plan to spend some time on the bargaining process; it can't be rushed. Allow time to listen to the clerk's story about the quality of the goods and to ask questions.

• Don't ask the price right away; instead discuss the attributes of the goods. When you do ask the price, don't reflect dismay or joy at the answer, just consider it a starting place for your discussions.

• Bury your ego so you will be able to admit to the clerk that you can't afford the item you like at the price quoted, and so that you can ask the clerk to help you figure out a way to help you buy your desired item.

- Be prepared to compliment the clerk, the store, and the goods, while remaining mildly disinterested. Call up your high school dramatics lessons for help in playing the role, if necessary.
- Spell out any limits that may affect your purchase or your time to bargain, such as needing to use a credit card, or wanting to ship the item. These limits may allow you to make counter-offers.
- Have counter-offers in mind, like buying two of the same item or paying cash, so the clerk will have some options in figuring out a deal that will work for both of you.
- Whenever an offer is accepted, the bargaining is over.
- Even if you don't make a deal, leave on good terms. For one thing, that's part of the fun of bargaining. For another, you could change your mind and return to the shop tomorrow.
- Don't second-guess your own purchase. Even if you come across a duplicate item later for half the price you paid, you paid what you thought the item was worth — so enjoy.

IN SUMMARY:

— Shop for items grown or made locally.
— Get receipts for whatever goods you buy.
— Don't expect super bargains at the duty-free shops.
— At overseas markets, learn how to bargain.

★ ★ ★
Travel Tool
★ ★ ★

BOOKS TO BROWSE

If you're interested in getting into the swing of recreational shopping, here are some books to browse.

Manston's Flea Markets series, each $9.95, from Travel Keys, P.O. Box 160691, Sacramento, CA 95816

Shopping in Exotic Places, by Ronald L. Krannich, Jo Reimer, Caryl Rae Krannich, $13.95 (plus $1.50 postage), Impact Publications, 10655 Big Oak Circle, Manassas, VA 22111 ☎ 703/361-7300.

How to Get Lost and Found series, $9.95 each (plus $2 postage), ORAFA Publishing Company, 1314 S. King St., Suite 1064, Honolulu, HI 96814.

Born to Shop series by Susan Schneider Thomas, $5.95 each, Bantam Books.

Travel Tool

★ ★ ★

SHOPPING FOR CLOTHES IN EUROPE

Clothing sizes are stated differently in America and Europe. But if you know what size American clothing you wear, use this chart to select comparable European sizes.

Do not rely on any chart — this one included — to guarantee a proper fit for your clothing. Always try on a garment before buying it.

MEN

SHOES

American	8	8 1/2	9	9 1/2	10	10 1/2	11
Continental	42	43	43	44	44	44	45

SUITS, SWEATERS, OVERCOATS

American	36	38	40	42	44	46	48
Continental	46	48	50	52	54	56	58

SHIRTS

American	14	14 1/2	15	15 1/2	16	16 1/2	17
Continental	36	37	38	39	40	41	42

WOMEN

SHOES

American	6	6 1/2	7	7 1/2	8	8 1/2	9
Continental	36	37	38	38	39	39	40

BLOUSES/SWEATERS

American	32	34	36	38	40	42	44
Continental	40	42	44	46	48	50	52

DRESSES/COATS/SUITS

American	8	10	12	14	16	18	20
Continental	36	38	40	42	44	46	48

CHAPTER 18

EATING AROUND

> ## It's a Large Part of the Joy When You Travel

W e'd gathered on the tour bus shortly after noon, ready to leave Munich, and began trading tales of our adventures in the Bavarian capital. Eating was on everyone's mind.

We drooled over memories of chocolaty Schwarzwald cakes, delicious *schweinehox* and *schnitzels,* sweet *strudels* and the liters of rich, dark beer that helped wash it all down. But the most enthusiastic were a young couple who'd found a very special restaurant 2,500 miles from home and wanted to share it with us:

On their very first day in Munich, they'd found a familiar restaurant and had a *viertel pfünder* — it tasted just like the ones at home. After that, for four days in Munich all they ate was that American delicacy, the *viertel pfünder* — MacDonald's Quarter-Pounder. They didn't have to survive on that funny German food.

We suppose this couple would have been comfortable almost anywhere in the world, for you can find Big Macs and Quarter Pounders in almost every civilized country, including the Soviet Union. Colonel Sanders chicken, too, as well as Cokes and Pepsis. And you can also get a well-done slab of beefsteak, so big that it hangs off the edge of your plate, almost anywhere.

But it seems to us that if you pass up the *rijstafel* in Amsterdam, the *vichyssoise* in Paris or the conch chowder in Nassau, you've missed a large part of the joy of traveling abroad. In this country, well-prepared chicken-fried steaks in Texas, Chesapeake Bay clambakes and Western family-style Basque

meals are local treats that are not well-known, yet alone dupli-
cated well, outside their regions.

Even sourdough bread doesn't taste as good outside San
Francisco, and any cheesesteak sandwich you eat outside of
Philadelphia is just not a Philly Cheesesteak.

In contrast, one of the worst meals we've ever eaten was a
Japanese steak dinner in Mexico. If nothing else, that taught us
to eat what the locals eat — after all, their chefs have spent a
lifetime getting it right.

EATING OUT ON A BUDGET

If you're on a cruise or a guided tour, most of your meals will
be pretty well planned — and pretty safe. You can arrange in
advance for special diets — kosher, low-salt, vegetarian and the
like. But on even the most expensive tour, you will still get a
chance to try the local fare.

And eating out doesn't have to be fancy. Gourmet meals, in
whatever country, are expensive, and most of us can't afford to
eat three of them every day.

One good way to economize is to cut back on other meals —
have juice and a roll for breakfast, if that's your habit at home,
or soup and a slab of cheese for lunch. But don't take economiz-
ing too far — an ample breakfast can keep you traveling in good
spirits all day.

Another way to conserve is to find out where the natives eat
— chances are the natives are on tighter budgets than you are.
Roadside stops and fast-food shops are not exclusive to America.
Other countries have their share of trattorias, coffee houses,
cafes, tavernas, tascas, tapas and other low-cost places where
light meals are served.

Unless your meals are prepaid, a hotel dining room is about
the most expensive place to eat an ordinary meal. Avoid breakfasts in your room, or lunch in the grill. Instead, take an
early-morning walk near your hotel and find out where the shop
clerks, the hotel employees or the white-collar workers eat their
breakfasts.

At lunch, watch for places where the working girls and the
delivery men eat — you can bet it won't be expensive. And,
especially overseas, you'll get to take part in some wonderful

local customs — the British pub lunch, for instance, or the German sausage break.

If you're driving, take along a picnic. Sandwiches and soft drinks purchased at a deli are cheaper than those bought at a sit-down coffee shop.

To hold down dinner costs, look for restaurants advertising early-bird specials, normally between 5 p.m. and 7 p.m. Though you'll find these everywhere, they're especially common in resort areas, where restaurants expect large late crowds but are usually empty earlier. You'll get the same meal, but it will be a few dollars cheaper.

If you're going to eat a full meal, steer clear of the á la carte restaurant, where everything from soup to nuts is priced separately. Less expensive is a complete dinner at a fixed price, especially if it's the daily special.

In Europe, many restaurants feature an economical daily tourist special at a fixed price. These will include a number of courses, plus taxes and tips.

The most expensive drink in foreign countries is hard liquor — even in countries like Scotland where some of the best hard liquor is made. Wine and beer are less costly, and every country has its special flavor. Coffee, tea and mineral water, of course, are the cheapest drinks of all.

LANGUAGE AND CUSTOMS

The toughest language barrier we ever encountered at a restaurant was in England, where most of the waiters are Yugoslav, Turkish, Vietnamese or the like — almost anything but English. Unable to communicate, we usually end up just pointing to menu items and hoping what comes is what we ordered. In other countries, ordering food is easier.

Except in France, don't be afraid you'll starve if you go to a restaurant where they speak a foreign language. France is the only place we remember where most menus weren't in English, as well as the native tongue and several other languages. And even in Paris, as we said, a little pigeon-French parlez-vous and a big smile will carry you a long way.

As for ordering wines, a sommelier is a sommelier everywhere — get his help. And just like trying the local food, we think drinking the local wine is part of the travel experience. We still smile at our friend, returning from France, who was outraged to find a Mondavi cabernet from the Napa Valley listed on a Paris *carte des vins* as a "foreign wine."

Of big help with the local language and customs are the *Marling Menu-Master* guides for France, Germany, Italy and Spain. The guides have English translations of a whole range of menu items, as well as information on types of cooking, tipping and local customs. You can find the Marling guides at most bookstores, or get a copy for $6.50 postpaid from The Traveller's Bookstore, 22 W. 52nd St., New York, NY 10019.

Although the listings aren't as extensive, the *Berlitz European Menu Reader* helps you with eating in 14 languages. *Simon and Schuster International Pocket Food Guide* is a menu decoder you can carry along in your pocket. These are also available at bookstores.

If you're very seriously into eating and cooking, shop the bookstore shelves for works of the individual countries you plan to visit, like Penelope Casas' *Foods and Wines of Spain*, or Alexis Lichine's *Guide to the Wines and Vineyards of France*.

FINDING A GOOD RESTAURANT

Finding a gourmet meal at a top-notch restaurant is easy. What's more difficult — and more rewarding — is finding a great meal at a restaurant that the locals like to keep to themselves.

For leading restaurants in any city — and some of the most expensive ones, too — check the guidebooks that rate them: AAA, Michelin and the like (see Chapter 4, Armchair Travel, for references). They're almost always reliable. Whether you end up with a four-star meal or a five-star meal at the Four Seasons in New York or Maxim's in Paris, you'll know you have eaten at a world-class restaurant. And you will have paid a world-class price, also.

For that class of restaurant, by the way, you have to make reservations, usually weeks in advance — no popping in at 5 p.m. and having the concierge make you 8 p.m. reservations. If your schedule is firm, ask your travel agent to make you reservations even before you leave home.

We prefer to steer clear of these kinds of places, though — with such grand expectations, we could only be disappointed. Instead, we like to find the sleepers, great little restaurants where the natives go, or the Maxim's of the future before the guidebooks discover them.

One great source we've used is the big-four travel magazines, especially *Travel & Leisure*, which often reviews local restaurants along with its travel articles. They're current and reliable.

Another good source is the hospitality person — desk clerk, concierge, bellman and the like. Tell them what kind of meal you're after and your price range, and half the time you will get a good recommendation. If you ask two or more, and the same restaurant name comes up, then you're starting to get a reliable fix.

In Las Vegas and Reno, for example, nobody knows more about local doings than the blackjack dealers. By asking the dealers this way, we found some wonderful restaurants:

"Other than right here at the hotel, what's the best Italian restaurant in town?" Or:

"If you were taking your family out for a good Italian meal, where would you go other than right here at the hotel?"

Of course, in Rome you don't want to ask for "a great Italian restaurant," or in Dijon for "a neat little French cafe." That's all they've got. So overseas, we just ask: "Where do local people like to eat dinner." That question works everywhere.

Get two or three restaurant names, check them against the phone-book ads to make sure they're the right kind of restaurants in decent neighborhoods, then check them once again with the desk clerk or hospitality desk just to be sure.

And a final word: If you're going to be spending a few days in a tourist area, don't just suppose you can always find a place to have your evening meal. We popped in hungry about 7 o'clock one night at the Cowboy Bar in Jackson, Wyo. — maybe the best steak house in the West — and found we couldn't get seated until 10:30. We got on the phone, but it was the same story at every other restaurant in town and at nearby Teton Village. We ended up with a hamburger at a fast-food joint.

The first day you're in a new location, plan where you want to eat and at what time, and make reservations for your stay. You can always call and cancel later if you change your plans.

EATING HEALTHY

One of our favorite signs is outside a roadhouse in the Minnesota northwoods: "Steaks, Chicken, Ribs, Worms, Night Crawlers." And we always wondered whether the crawlers were prepared steamed or fried.

Yes, you do take chances of ending up with an upset stomach whenever you eat out — even in your home town and at Midwest roadhouses. But as Peter Greenberg, the *Savvy Traveler* columnist, wrote, "Given the choice between the possibility of an upset stomach in Rome and Bangkok vs. New York and Chicago, I'll take Italy and Thailand every time."

A 1987 British survey reported that stomach problems account for about 60 percent of travelers' illnesses. The highest risk was to travelers to Egypt, India, Turkey, Kenya, Tunisia, Morocco and the U.S.S.R. The lowest risk to travelers was in the Netherlands, Belgium, Ireland and West Germany. The U.S. and Mexico came out somewhere in the middle.

In Chapter 20, we list some precautions you should take to guard your health when you eat out — don't drink the water, peel your own fruit, avoid food that's been standing around and so forth. But don't be paranoid about it.

Wherever you travel in America or abroad, you have to eat somewhere. So we think you should enjoy it.

IN SUMMARY:

— Eating the local foods is part of the travel experience.
— To economize, cut back on breakfast or lunch, eat where the locals eat have a picnic or try "earlybird specials."
— Most restaurants overseas have English-language menus.
— Look for the great little restaurants the locals like to keep to themselves.
— Be health- and diet-conscious, but don't let precautions spoil your trip.

Travel Tool

★ ★ ★

WHAT'S GOOD FOR YOU

While we believe that travelers who stick with strict diets miss lots of the fun of eating out in a foreign atmosphere, there's no harm in being health conscious. And there's no law that says you have to eat everything on your plate. In its pamphlet *Healthy Eating Away from Home*, the makers of Sweet 'N Low and other foods for weight-loss dieters list these guidelines to follow when dining out:

Chinese — Choose steamed or lightly stir-fried entrees without salt or MSG, brown rice (not white rice to which soy sauce has been added) instead of white. Avoid fried foods, fried rice and noodles; skip sweet and sour dishes.

French — Request that sauces be served on the side. Opt for chicken, veal, lean beef or seafood prepared in classic stews or light sauces. Avoid au gratin dishes, rich sauces such as bearnaise, bechamel and hollandaise.

Italian — Select pastas with tomato, marinara or red clam sauce, rather than butter, cream, heavy cheese or rich meat sauces; pasta primavera with vegetables is also good. Avoid veal scallopine or parmigiana, fried eggplant with cheese.

Japanese — Ideal for the dieter are sushi and sashimi and pickled vegetables. Entrees made with tofu are excellent. Ask for sauces on the side; use sparingly.

Mexican — Go easy on tortilla chips. Order baked, not fried, Mexican dishes; seviche (marinated fish); shrimp or chicken tostados on cornmeal tortillas (not fried). Avoid refried beans (high in fat). Ask that sour cream and cheese be served on the side.

New American Cuisine — Choose from native American foods such as gumbo, Cajun blackened redfish; broiled catfish; Tex-Mex fajitas, thin-sliced meat with flour tortillas; black beans; pizza; blue cornmeal; chili peppers and mushrooms. Avoid deep-fried fish or chicken and French fries, extra cheese on pizza (add more vegetables). Quiche may seem like a healthy dish, but it can be laden with eggs, cream and high-fat cheese.

Seafood restaurants — Select halibut, sea bass, swordfish, red snapper, salmon, scallops or other such fish. Have it broiled, steamed, grilled or baked with wine or lemon juice and fresh herbs. Avoid deep-fried seafood with breading or batter coating, lobster with melted butter.

Steakhouse — A good choice, since food is most often prepared to order. Choose lean entrees like London broil, filet mignon, round and flank steaks. Specify broiling without additional fat or salt. Order baked potato with yogurt instead of sour cream. Avoid French fries, rich salad dressings, BBQ ribs with rich sauces and oversize steaks.

For a copy of the pamphlet *Healthy Eating Away from Home*, send 25 cents to Cumberland Packing Corp., 60 Flushing Ave., Dept. TMT, Brooklyn, NY 11205. Cumberland is the maker of Sweet 'N Low® ,Butter Buds® and Nu-Salt®.

Travel Tool

★ ★ ★

DECODING THE MENU

Here's how to decipher some common menu items when you're traveling abroad:

English	French	German	Italian	Spanish
bread	pain	Brot	pane	pan
beef	boeuf	Rindfleisch	manzo	carne de res
lamb	agneau	Lammfleish	agnello	cordero
pork	porc	Schweinefleisch	carne di maiale	cerdo
veal	veau	Kalbfleisch	vitello	ternera
chicken	poulet	Huhn	pollo	pollo
duck	canard	Ente	anitra	pato
fish	poisson	Fisch	pesce	pescado
water	eau	Wasser	acqua	agua
red wine	vin rouge	Rotwein	vino rosso	vino tinto
white wine	vin blanc	Weisswein	vino bianco	vino blanco
rare	saignant	roh	poco cotto	poco hecho
medium	á point	halbdurch	cottura media	medio hecho
well-done	bien cuit	durchgebraten	ben cotto	bien hecho

CHAPTER 19

TIPPING

| It Can Make Good Things Happen for You |

To Insure Promptness — that's what "T.I.P." is supposed to stand for. But over the years, the custom of rewarding people for attentive service has changed so dramatically that even veteran travelers are unsure of how much to leave.

In some parts of the world, cash gifts, including tips, are interpreted as insults or bribes. In other places, "gratuities" (read "tips") are added to bills automatically, so there is no longer any pretense that you're leaving a reward for good service. In many service establishments nowadays, owners pay minimum wages with the understanding that tips will boost the service person's income to a fairly decent level.

This occurs at casinos, especially, where under-salaried dealers often bring home 60-to-70 percent of their income in tips.

WHY TIP, ANYHOW?

Why should you leave a tip at all for a waiter you'll never see again at an establishment you'll never return to? Well, among travelers it should be a kind of social compact. The reason your service was good was probably because a previous traveler rewarded it with a tip. The tip you leave may ensure that the next traveler gets good service.

And if you'll be around awhile — returning to that same restaurant, staying at the hotel for several days or on a cruise or guided tour for a few weeks, you may be surprised how adequate tipping makes good things happen for you.

The problem is figuring out what's adequate. We can think of no other aspect of travel we have disagreed on over the years as often as on the amount of tip to leave — which service person has earned a reward and which one hasn't. And how much. The notion of handing out a sum of money we've computed on a fixed percentage like robots goes against our grain. Especially when the "thank-you" money is going to a person whose work has been only average — someone whose training and pay should be the responsibility of the employer, not the guest.

On the other hand, we all want to do what's right, and to be liked and appreciated. The idea of being chased down a street by a waiter who wants to return a small tip with a sarcastic comment like, "You need this more than I do" — which happened to us once after a meal at an over-rated restaurant in Chicago — is not appealing.

When we tip, we like to give a message — that the service has been superb (20 percent of the check, or more) or that it's been lousy (20 cents or thereabouts). If you don't leave a tip at all, an incompetent waiter might think that here are people who simply never tip anywhere. So we always leave at least few pennies to indicate that, yes, we always tip, and no, this kind of service didn't rate much of one.

We don't mean to shrug off the subject or leave it with advice like, "Tip when you feel the service deserves it." People from all segments of the travel industry say tipping is the single most frequent subject they're asked about.

On the other hand, there's no way we can tell you how much to tip when we don't know whether you had to wait for 20 minutes for a menu or haven't seen whether the waiter acted as if he were doing you a favor. You have to know local customs and use your own sense of fair play when determining the right amount to tip.

If you feel you need some advice to learn the local customs, there's always an expert around. In a hotel, the concierge will know what's appropriate for nearly every occasion, both inside the hotel and out; on a ship, the cruise director or purser can help.

A good book that covers every tipping situation we can think of is Nancy Star's *International Guide to Tipping* ($5.95, Berkeley Books). It's small enough to take along and use for reference.

Wherever you are, never hold out a handful of coins and have someone select his own tip. And even though many travel writers recommend doing it, we also avoid asking the person to be tipped how much he should get. That's something like asking your grandchildren how much they want for a birthday gift.

TIPS ON TIPPING

There are some basic rules of thumb that you can take with you everywhere to help you make your decisions:

Know the country. When doing your homework about the countries you'll be visiting, ask about the laws of the land. For example, in countries like China and Russia, tips are looked on as bribes and could land you in serious trouble. In other countries, like Nigeria or the Philippines, tips are considered bribes — but legally accepted bribes. And in some other countries, like Japan, tipping is not yet the accepted custom.

In some countries — Mexico with its Value Added Tax (VAT) and America with its sales tax — people often compute their tips based on a total that includes the tax. Check your bill carefully before computing your tip. It's a waste to tip 15 percent on $3 worth of taxes when the total bill was $15.

Know what service is. Each of us has a pretty good idea when we're being abused by a waiter or a cab driver. We've established a standard of what we call good service. Apply that standard fairly. Don't penalize the waiter if the cook has prepared you a raw steak when you ordered yours well done. But do penalize the waiter if he refuses to return it to the kitchen or returns it with something less than grace.

Know the company policy. Some companies such as hotels, restaurants and cruiselines have adopted "no-tipping" policies. One such is the Holland America lines. Even on these ships, however, most passengers will leave small tips for the room steward and waiter for services performed.

At some leading resorts in America and at restaurants throughout much of Europe (Portugal excepted), tips are included in your bill's total. So to offer a 15 percent tip on top of a 15 percent gratuity would be wasteful — yet many unaware Americans do just that. If you've had astonishing service, you might want to leave an additional 3- to 5- percent on top of the built-in 15 percent.

Know the house practices. Many service people split their tips with fellow workers. Restaurant waiters commonly split tips with their busboys, and sometimes with the chef and the maitre d'. Cocktail servers split with the bartender. In casinos, every dealer shares in the "toke" or tip you give your dealer.

If you want to reward somebody in addition to the one who served you directly, ask discreetly whether that person shares in the tips. If you tip everyone in sight, you could end up leaving behind 30 or 40 percent — too much, no matter how good the service.

Know the currency-exchange rate. Familiarize yourself with the cash of the country by asking your bank or money-changer to give you $1 in foreign coins. That way you can become comfortable with the coins and what $1 looks like in the currency you'll be dealing with. Also ask how acceptable American money is in the country. If it is commonly accepted for goods and services, 10 or 15 dollar bills can be very helpful in dealing with people who go out of their way to make your trip enjoyable.

Know yourself. Be willing not to tip — and deal with the gaff if it comes. Tips should not be blackmail. If you have not received the service you want or expect, do not feel obliged to hand out money anyway.

We do think it means more when we can explain to the maitre d' or manager that we have had poor service and describe what was wrong. And if we've had a particularly good experience, we often write notes when we get home. The notes seem to mean more than money.

SOME TIPPING GUIDELINES

Here are some common travel-tipping situations:
• Airport limo drivers — Give $1-$2 per person in your party, depending on whether the driver has loaded and unloaded the baggage.
• Baggage handlers/bellhops — Give $1 per bag.
• Bartenders — Leave 50 cents to $1 per round when you settle up your tab.

• Buffets/cafeterias — Only 5 to 10 percent. After all, mostly you've served yourself.

• Cabin steward or attendant — Leave $2 per day per person, more if you are traveling deluxe. Envelopes are often provided by the ship to be used the last night of a cruise. If it is a longer cruise — a month or more — tip every two weeks or so.

• Casino dealers — A tip or "toke," as it's called in towns like Atlantic City and Las Vegas, is generally expected when you've had a good time or have been winning. Even though dealers customarily pool all their tips, they tend to take tipping very personally — as a compliment or a slight. Limit tips during play — unless you've hit it big — and then share a dollar or two with the dealer as you leave. Instead of tipping, some players play money for the dealer, on top of their regular bet — usually about half of what a normal tip would be. If you lose, the dealer loses; if you win the dealer gets double. If you're a big winner, your tip should reflect that. Big losers are not expected to tip much. And sour dealers who don't make much effort to conduct a fun table shouldn't be rewarded, either.

• Concierge — This person can be your lifesaver — finding you tickets, giving you directions, recommending restaurants or other attractions. In America, most concierges or hotel hosts are on salary and do not expect tips. In Europe and elsewhere overseas, however, the concierge is often a freelancer working for commissions from the shows or restaurants you're sent to, and tips are accepted. If your use of the concierge is about average, the tip should be $5 to $7 when you check out. If you are asking for additional help, like mailing packages or tracking down scarce show tickets, increase the tip to thank the concierge for time spent.

• Maitre d'hotel — If you're unexpectedly given an excellent table during peak hours, $2 to $5 makes a nice thank-you when you leave. If you're after scarce seats to a sold-out nightclub show, a huge tip to the maitre d' often will get you in. No matter how crowded the room, maitres d' always hold back a few seats for VIPs. A $50 tip makes you a VIP.

• Personal services (hairdresser, masseuse, manicurist) — Follow your practice from home — unless home means a small town or your hair is done by the owner.

• Table captain — This is the person who takes your order in a fine restaurant. If that's all he does, there's no need to be particularly generous. If he creates your salad, cooks your dinner, decants your wine and flambés your dessert, you should consider leaving 5 to 10 percent.

• Theater usher — A customary tip in Europe is the equivalent 50 cents.

• Tour escort — For the escort who stays with you throughout your tour, $1-$2 per day per person is in order, if it's been a good tour. Leave more if the escort has done a number of special services for you.

• Tour guides/drivers — Shorter day-trips are usually rewarded with $1-$2 per person for the guide, and an extra 75 cents to $1.50 for the driver. For longer tours, the rate should increase to $1.50 to $3 per day per person for the guide, with an equivalent increase for the driver. The guide and the driver often share tips.

• Waiter (restaurant) — The customary 10 percent (lunch) to 20 percent (dinner) is good around the world, except at restaurants where a gratuity is automatically added to your tab or where tipping is forbidden.

• Waiter (resort or cruiseship) — Leave $2 to $3 per day if service is not included in your bill.

• Washroom/locker-room attendant — Tip 25 to 50 cents, if some service, like a hand-towel, is provided.

• Wine steward — Depending on the quality of the restaurant and the quality of the advice, tip 7 to 10 percent of the cost of the wine. On a ship, the tip should be given when the wine is brought to your table — not at the end of the cruise.

IN SUMMARY:

— Be familiar with the local currency to avoid under- or over-tipping.
— Find out the local customs for tipping — they vary all over the world.
— Be fair when you tip — reward good service.
— But don't reward bad service with a good tip.

CHAPTER 20

TO YOUR HEALTH

Planning Ahead Can Save Your Trip

George and his Missus had been looking forward to the vacation for the best part of a year, and the trip had been going just fine. But now George is confined to his hotel room with a case of diarrhea while everyone else is touring the French countryside. There's nothing in his kit to cure it, and George is too embarrassed to ask a stranger behind the counter of a drug store, in a strange language, what he might do about it.

Could he have prevented the problem?

No doubt — with some planning ahead.

Although the Centers for Disease Control in Atlanta has estimated that the average traveler has a one-in-five chance of getting sick and other estimates range up to twice that likelihood, you can keep the odds on your side by doing your homework and taking common-sense precautions.

Doctors on cruise ships, for example, report the two most frequent medical complaints of passengers are sunburn and forgetfulness — many forget to bring their medication. Both problems are easily prevented by planning.

That doesn't mean planning will help you avoid something completely unexpected, like a broken hip, but planning ahead will permit you to enjoy your trip with more confidence.

PRE-TRIP PLANNING

Part of your vacation planning should include anticipating problems. For instance, if you have difficulty with breathing, don't plan a trip to a high-altitude area.

Health questions to consider when making travel plans include:

• Does the tour provide you enough time to recover from jet lag or other travel exhaustion?

• If you have walking or respiratory problems, do the attractions include endless stairways or other access difficulties?

• Do you have the energy to deal with the travel schedule as planned (up early every day, a different hotel every night, long hours on sightseeing buses)?

• Does the destination have built-in problems for you, such as climate, lack of sanitation facilities or medical treatment facilities?

GETTING YOUR CHECKUPS

Once you've selected your destinations, make appointments with your dentist and doctor.

The dental appointment should be about four weeks before departure. That way, if you need work done, like having a filling replaced, you will have time to get comfortable with the results before traveling too far. Don't fly for at least 12 hours after fillings, root canals or extractions — the atmospheric pressure can cause pain.

Visit your doctor about six weeks before you leave, and bring along a copy of your itinerary and all information you've collected about the places you'll be touring. The information should include details about altitude and climate, including average temperatures and humidity, what vaccinations are required and if an AIDS-antibody test is needed. Use the information to discuss any limits the doctor may feel are important for your health, and any alterations in your medication that may be caused by the places you will be visiting. For example, recent heart patients might want to plan extra rest periods when visiting hot and humid locations. And high altitudes can change the way certain drugs affect you.

258

Diabetic travelers should work with their doctors to map out programs to prevent problems. Such a program would allow for eating whatever foods are available at your destination, planning for the effects of increased exercise, and briefing your travel companion on how to deal with a diabetic coma.

There are more than 100 countries where diseases like malaria, yellow fever and cholera exist. Vaccinations are mandatory for cholera and yellow fever, and you'll be asked to show an International Vaccination Certificate, a yellow card attesting to the date and type of vaccination you've had, signed by the physician.

Many physicians will recommend that anyone going to a developing country should have typhoid, gamma globulin and polio immunizations, as well.

Malaria is common in many parts of the Caribbean, Mexico, South America, Asia and Africa. A World Malaria Risk Chart of countries where malaria is found is available at no cost from the International Association for Medical Assistance to Travelers (IAMAT), 417 Center St., Lewiston, NY 14092; ☎ 716/754-4883. Many physicians recommend weekly doses of chloroquine as a preventative, though not for patients with gastro-intestinal problems.

In addition to any shots you may need for your destinations, ask your physician for a written, generic prescription of any medications you're using, along with the dosage. The prescription should include a short physician's memo listing any specific medical problems that trouble you, including allergies. If you don't know what your blood type is, have that information added to the doctor's memo. If you have been a cardiac patient, carry a copy of your most recent electrocardiogram and a medical history. Take two copies of all medical data and keep each in a different place, such as your wallet and your carry-on luggage.

If you wear eyeglasses or contact lenses, plan to carry a copy of your prescription and an extra pair of glasses, as well as supplies for cleaning glasses and lenses. Remember that if a country's water supply is not considered safe for drinking, it probably should not be used to clean contact lenses.

Carry artificial teardrops and use them in dry conditions such as long airplane flights, high-altitude locations, cold weather or arid areas.

259

List contacts on your medical-emergency wallet card; medical personnel will then know to remove your lenses during treatment.

PACKING FOR HEALTH

We'd arrived on the plane at Munich with a tour party that included two wonderful ladies traveling together. Though they'd kept hand-baggage with them, one of the ladies had packed her medicines in her suitcase. Unhappily, her bag was flying on to Vienna.

One of the medicines in the lady's suitcase was to control her high blood pressure. For four days — while the airline was finding her suitcase — she had to stay around the hotel, unable to keep up with the tour's heavy sightseeing schedule. Of course, her companion spent much of that time with her, also missing many of the pleasures of the Bavarian capital.

It could have been avoided had the lady packed her medicine in hand-luggage that stayed with her. For air travel, that means carry-on luggage. In addition, wise travelers carry a couple of days' supply of required medications in their pockets or purses.

Take along a supply of prescription medications that will be adequate for the length of your trip. Keep pills in the prescription containers given to you by the pharmacist. That way, you will prevent any interaction of the drugs, and by keeping them in the original bottles and boxes, you'll head off disputes with customs about bringing drugs into a foreign country. Plastic bottles are preferred, but if glass bottles are necessary, put them inside a self-sealing plastic bag.

If you have a condition like diabetes or epilepsy that can render you unexpectedly unconscious, wear or carry medical-identification information. You can get a tag from Medic-Alert, Box 1009, Turlock, CA 95381 (☎ 800/344-3226; in California 209/668-3333); or Health Enterprises, Inc., 15 Spruce St., North Attleboro, MA 02760 (☎ 800/833-4243 or 508/695-0727).

Those taking Saga Holidays tours can order their medical-record data on a microfilm chip sealed in a wallet-size plastic card. In emergencies, though, medical authorities warn, you may not be able to have these chips read in time to be of any help, especially in third-world countries.

Diabetics should pack a couple of candy bars along with an adequate supply of monitoring paraphernalia and disposable syringes.

Heart patients carrying nitroglycerin should keep the medication in a sealed brown bottle. Remember to remove the cotton, since it can absorb the ingredients. Keep nitroglycerin away from temperature extremes.

Even if you are totally healthy, it's a good idea to carry along a well-stocked first-aid kit. Helpful items include:
- Aspirin
- Antihistamine-decongestants
- Sunscreens
- Anti-diarrhea preparations
- Antiseptic
- Contact lens paraphernalia
- Bandages or Band-Aids of different sizes
- Anti-motion sickness medications
- Laxative
- Antacid tablets
- Skin cream
- Water purifiers
- Insect repellent.

MOTION SICKNESS

Getting there can be very uncomfortable for some 21 million Americans who suffer from motion sickness, with symptoms that include nausea, cold sweats, pallor and vomiting. But there are ways to limit such discomfort.

Stay where the chances of unusual or sudden motion are kept to a minimum — for example, in the middle of a ship at sea. Don't look out the porthole or fix your gaze on any object that's swaying, like a chandelier. Stay in places where there is adequate ventilation. Avoid alcohol and heavy meals, and be properly rested.

There are many anti-motion remedies, but they can cause side effects such as drowsiness or headaches. Work with your physician to find the best remedy for you.

Among available prescription devices is a Transderm Scop, a dime-sized medicated adhesive patch worn behind the ear. It uses the skin to deliver a drug called scopolamine directly into the wearer's bloodstream. This patch should be used with caution because it can interact with other drugs you may be taking. If there's any doubt, check with your physician or a pharmacist before using it.

Transderm Scops — commonly called "seasick patches" — are usually available for the asking to passengers aboard ships.

Another anti-motion sickness technique is autogenic feedback, a hypnosis-like procedure that helps you control such bodily functions as blood flow, heart rate and respiration rate that contribute to motion sickness. Details about autogenic feedback training are available from scientists specializing in biofeedback. Ask your doctor how to find one.

HOW TO STAY AIRBORNE AND HEALTHY

The cabin of an airliner is not a healthy environment.

The artificial pressure inside an airplane is equivalent to that at about an 8,000-foot altitude, and it's just air — no moisture. In addition, you sit for long hours in cramped seats, drink more than you ought to and eat one or more meals that can triple your daily intake of calories.

You can order diet meals, vegetarian meals, salt-free meals or kosher meals instead of the regular airline fare if you do it when you buy your ticket.

You can hold down your drinking — alcohol is a diuretic, and dries you out even more.

You can bring a moisturizing lotion to lubricate dry skin.

And you can walk around and do other exercises to head off stiffness.

Many travelers find the long sit on plane, train, bus or in the car harmful to their backs. To alleviate any damage, put a pillow against your lower back. If a pillow isn't available, use what is — a coat, a small blanket — or even your arm. Get up every half-hour or so and walk around the plane.

Periodic walking up and down the aisles is also good for anyone suffering from phlebitis. Avoid wearing clothes — particularly stockings or panty hose — that bind or impede circulation.

Exercising in your seat is a good idea, too. Two airlines offer free brochures describing in-flight exercises. *Medical Hints for Travel Abroad* is available by sending a self-addressed long envelope to Dept. MT, Lufthansa German Airlines, 240 Stockton St., San Francisco, CA 94108. *Exercise in the Chair* is available free from Scandinavian Airlines System, 138-02 Queens Blvd., Jamaica, NY 11435.

HAZARDS OF FLYING

Flying offers special hazards if you have flu, a cold or allergies. You can develop painful sinus and ear problems as a result of cabin pressure changes. If you must fly, take an oral decongestant an hour before your plane comes down, and also perform what doctors call the "modified Valsalva maneuver." You call it "popping your ears" — pinching your nose, closing your mouth and trying to breathe outward.

Those with these following medical problems should not fly at all, according to the American Medical Association:

Recent heart attack or stroke, severe high blood pressure, severe heart disease, pneumothorax (air outside the lungs), cysts of the lung or any acute lung disease, acute sinusitis or middle-ear infections, recent abdominal surgery, acute diverticulitis or ulcerative colitis, acute esophageal or intestinal viruses, epilepsy, recent skull fracture or brain tumor, severe anemia, sickle cell disease, hemophilia with active bleeding, recent eye surgery or wiring of the jaw.

And if you have chronic heart or lung problems, ask the airline to have supplemental oxygen available during the flight.

BEATING JET LAG

What could be worse than finding yourself in the city of your dreams — and dreaming the hours away because of jet lag?

Jet lag mostly is caused by the difference between your body's clock and the clock at your destination. You leave New York at 6 p.m., scheduled to arrive in London at 6 the next morning. During the flight, you have a leisurely meal, watch the movie and sip a drink. Around midnight, you're ready for a night's sleep. But by then the sun is up and you're within an hour of arriving. Somewhere, your body has lost five hours. While bright-eyed Londoners are just getting out and about, ready to face the day, you are ready for nothing but eight hours of shut-eye. Worse, after you get it, you wake up bright-eyed in the middle of the afternoon, and can't get to sleep that night to save your soul. Sometimes, the process can go on for three days before you get adjusted.

A recent study showed that nine out of 10 long-distance east-west travelers suffered some form of jet lag — 45 percent of them with severe symptoms.

The trick is, before you go, slowly fool your body into thinking it's already there.

By coping with the problem before it occurs, you'll prevent irritability and excessive fatigue, and you'll be better able to make decisions and enjoy the sights.

If you're crossing more than three time zones, schedule the trip in stages, with a layover between legs. If that's not possible, plan your trip so you arrive in the evening. If the airline schedules don't permit this choice — and on most west-to-east flights they don't — try the jet-lag diet that will help you reset your body clock.

Here's how the jet-lag diet works:

Four days before you leave, eat high-protein foods at breakfast and lunch. For dinner, choose mostly carbohydrates. Drink coffee only from 3 p.m. to 5 p.m.

Three days before you leave, eat lightly, keeping your total calories and carbohydrates down and again limiting your coffee drinking to between 3 and 5 p.m.

Two days before departure, repeat the high-protein breakfast and lunch and carbohydrate dinner. The day before you leave, again eat lightly.

If possible, pair the jet-lag diet with changes in your sleeping schedule. For example, travelers planning to fly east to west — to San Francisco, Hawaii or the Orient — should begin getting up a bit later for each of the three days before departure. Those going west to east — to New York, London or the rest of Europe — should wake a bit earlier each day.

On the plane, avoid alcoholic beverages, sleep as much as possible until it's breakfast time at your destination, and then rise and shine and eat hearty!

To get to sleep on the plane, relax. On a long flight, take off your shoes; some airlines provide slippers for passengers on long overseas flights. And wear loose, comfortable clothing — sweatsuits are becoming more common on airliners these days.

AT EASE WITH THE ELEMENTS

The elements you cope with easily at home — heat, humidity, cold, insects, altitude, sun — can lead to trouble far from home. If you're aware of the dangers, it will go a long way toward helping you prevent problems.

For example, if you are accustomed to living near sea level and will be traveling to an altitude around 8,000 feet, try to make the ascent slowly over a two- or three-day period. Avoid strenuous activities the first few days, and you may avoid symptoms of headache, shortness of breath, lightheadedness, nausea or other flu-like complaints.

Minimize the dangers of heat exhaustion by drinking plenty of fluids, avoiding the noon-day sun, wearing a head covering, and getting plenty of sleep.

If you have allergies, stay in air-conditioned hotels, keep car and other windows closed early in the day or when traveling through areas with lots of vegetation, and don't collect flowers.

To avoid attracting insects, don't wear perfume or perfumed cosmetics. Wear clothing that covers arms and legs. Carry insect repellent and use it on both body and clothing. Put nets over beds and windows in tropical areas. And don't scratch bites.

TOURISTS' REVENGE

Whether you're actually suffering that awful combination of diarrhea, cramps, chills and fever called "Montezuma's Revenge," or just reacting from the effects of new places and new foods, digestive problems are probably the single most-common ailment affecting travelers.

Here are several ways to avoid stomach problems:

• Eat familiar foods — especially at the beginning of the trip — and eat at familiar hours. Save exotic foods for later in the journey when you are better acclimated. Try to avoid big meals or experimenting with strange foods late at night.

- Don't overindulge — with either food or drink.
- If you're prone to constipation, drink lots of bottled water.
- If you're prone to indigestion, carry your favorite non-prescription remedy, like Maalox or Tums.
- If you're prone to stress, set aside some time each day to relax quietly with eyes closed and feet up.

To head off diarrhea:

- Don't eat from sidewalk stands. Especially, avoid raw fruits unless you, personally, peel the fruit. If the skin of the fruit is broken, don't eat it.
- Avoid locally bottled, non-carbonated water — especially if it is served uncapped. Drink name-brand soft drinks, beer or wine out of bottles. Drink beverages that have been made with boiled water, like tea and coffee. Avoid ice cubes.
- Avoid raw greens and things like tossed salads outside of northern Europe.
- Avoid fresh milk in developing countries or the tropics unless it has been boiled. Avoid fresh cheese.
- Don't eat perishables such as custards, creams, foods made with mayonnaise or fresh salads.
- Brush your teeth with bottled, carbonated water.
- Avoid eating raw or undercooked fish and meat.

If you're going somewhere you know the water is bad, take along Halozone tablets, which you can buy at any drugstore. You can also boil it. Another way to make the water safe is to put two drops of liquid laundry bleach (like Clorox) or a few drops of tincture of iodine in a quart of water and let it stand for a half hour. If you can taste the bleach or the iodine, the water will probably be safe. If you can't taste the dosage, add more.

If you follow all these precautions and still get tourists' revenge, here's what to do:

If your diarrhea is mild (up to two loose bowel movements in an eight-hour period), take a remedy such a Lomotil, Pepto-Bismol, Kaopectate or Pargel. You can buy any of these without prescription at pharmacies in most foreign countries. The diarrhea should stop in about a day.

If your diarrhea is more severe (more than three loose bowel movements in eight hours), consider taking an antibiotic such as tetracycline. That's a potent prescription drug, and don't use it unless your doctor has given you the all-clear.

266

Diarrhea is extremely dehydrating, causing you to feel weak. You need to replace vital fluids — but water will not do the trick alone. The Centers for Disease Control recommend this recipe to help (if you are diabetic, check this with your physician before using):

In one glass put 8 ounces of orange juice, 1/2 tsp. honey, corn syrup or sugar, and a pinch of salt.

In a second glass, put 8 ounces carbonated or boiled water and 1/4 tsp. baking soda.

Drink alternately from each glass.

If you have trouble finding those ingredients, another, simple recipe you can prepare is 1 tsp. salt, 1 tsp. baking soda, 4 tsp. sugar, 1 qt. bottled water.

Supplement this with other liquids like hot tea or boiled water. Avoid solid foods and milk — foods like plain rice or rice meal are okay.

MUSEUM FEET

Your feet are also prone to damage when traveling. The best advice when trying to prevent damage to them is: don't overdo.

Many people underestimate how much walking will be required on a trip. It's better to assume there will be a lot and take along at least two pairs of very comfortable shoes — then alternate wearing them. Never take new shoes when traveling. Before you leave home, take care of corns and calluses. Take — and wear — appropriate foot coverings when walking on the beach and wading in the sea. Coral wounds and jellyfish stings can be painful surprises, but a cheap pair of tennis shoes — light enough to swim in — will protect your feet against almost any peril of the sea.

Baby your feet at the end of each day. Do simple massages, such as using your hand to gently squeeze your toes and bend them back and forth. Or make a "fist" with your foot and bend the toes inward slowly. Alternate feet and repeat several times. When barefooted, interlace your fingers with your toes and squeeze gently. Soak your feet in a mixture of 2 teaspoons of Epsom salts in warm water.

If there is swelling, apply ice compresses.

If a blister has broken, paint it with antiseptic and cover with a gauze bandage. Then try to keep the walking pressure off it for a day or two.

DEADLY SUNSHINE

Whether it's sunshine on the beach or on ski slopes, it can be dangerous. And it can accelerate the aging process. Ultraviolet rays help destroy the connective tissue that keeps the skin tight; when it breaks down, wrinkles occur. So when confronting the sun on either sand or snow, take it easy:

• Stay out of the high-noon sun.

• Use a sunscreen. If you've had recent plastic surgery, avoid the sun altogether for at least a year and then use a No. 18 or No. 19 screen. If you're taking antibiotics, barbiturates, diabetic drugs, some kinds of anti-malaria pills or diuretics, your skin is likely to be more susceptible to the sun.

• Use a good pair of sunglasses made of optical glass that allow through between 15 and 35 percent of visible light.

• Wear light-colored, loose-fitting clothes made of natural fibers.

• Wear a hat that protects your head and neck.

• Avoid wearing perfumes or colognes in the sun. Many have an ingredient called bergamot that can increase sensitivity to the sun.

• If you have suffered a sunburn, use a moisturizing cream, drink water, eat lightly, rest.

If you are irritable, sluggish, tired, have a fast pulse, have stomach cramps, and are perspiring heavily, you may be suffering from heat exhaustion. Sponge your body with cool water, and drink a liquid.

Heat stroke is an extreme form in which you stop sweating, feel feverish and have a fast pulse. If you get these symptoms, reduce your body temperature quickly by sponging with cold water or alcohol. Get medical help.

FINDING HELP

Even the best-planned trip can result in problems — a twisted ankle, exhaustion, an infected scratch, or strained back.

While most hotel physicians are well-trained, they may not speak English or may not have the specialized training required for your problem.

To find an all-night drug-store or pharmacy, call the local police; they are most likely to have a list of those operating 24 hours.

Before you leave, get a list of English-speaking physicians in the areas you plan to visit. Such a list is available through U.S. consulates or the International Association for Medical Assistance to Travelers (IAMAT) 417 Center St., Lewiston, NY 14092; ☎ 716/754-4883.

If you join Access America (see next section, Health Insurance), you'll have a 24-hour hotline wherever you travel that will help you find an English-speaking doctor.

American consular offices are generally knowledgeable about doctors or hospitals in their service areas. The American embassy in the capital city of the country you are visiting should have a 24-hour emergency phone number to call for help.

Full-service university teaching hospitals are another good source of English-speaking doctors and can offer a wide range of medical services. For emergencies in this country or overseas, look for the international symbol for "hospital," a white "H" printed on a blue background.

The U. S. State Department's Overseas Citizen's Emergency Center, Washington, DC 20520, offers various publications to help alert you to medical problems you may encounter while traveling overseas. For example, the center issues warning about health and safety problems, such as disease outbreaks. Advisories are available by calling the center at ☎ 202/632-5225 or by writing to the address above.

The Superintendent of Documents, Government Printing Office, Washington, DC 20402, also offers information, including leaflets called *Tips for Travelers*, with a separate leaflet for each foreign country. Also available at no charge through the documents office is *Travel Tips for Senior Citizens* and a 32-page booklet, *Your Trip Abroad*, that deals with carrying prescription narcotic drugs. Each publication costs $1.

In the case of a genuine emergency, medical dispensaries at U.S. Armed Forces bases may provide outpatient service to U.S. civilians. But be prepared to prove it's a real emergency.

HEALTH INSURANCE

Check your medical insurance before you leave to find out what coverage it provides when you travel overseas. In most cases, you'll be expected to pay for hospital care in cash or traveler's checks. But your insurance may reimburse you, provided you have adequate documentation.

Medicare does not cover overseas medical services, although some supplementary policies may. After checking your coverage, you may want to have your agent provide you with a short-term policy for such travel services as medical expenses, trip cancellation, accidental injury and lost baggage.

Another option is a supplementary policy for travelers. An example of such a policy for both foreign and domestic travel is issued by Access America, a subsidiary of Blue Cross and Blue Shield. Through its 24-hour hotline, Access America will put you in touch with doctors, dentists and pharmacies. The policy pays hospitalization anywhere up to $10,000 per person or $20,000 per family, and provides for medical evacuation back to the United States, if you need it. Access America helps with lost documents, passports and airline tickets. The policy will provide bail if you get into trouble overseas, and it covers against auto accidents, trip cancellation and baggage loss. Access America can be reached at 600 Third Avenue, Box 807, New York, NY 10163.

Others offering overseas health insurance policies include:

• The Travelers Insurance Companies, Travel Pak, One Tower Square, Hartford, CT 06115.

• International SOS Assistance, Inc., One Neshaminy Interplex, Trevose, PA 19047.

• WorldCare Travel Assistance Association Inc., 2000 Pennsylvania Ave.N.W., #7600, Washington, DC 20006.

• TravMed, P.O. Box 10623, Towson, MD 21204.

• Travel Assistance International, 1133 15th St., N.W., Suite 4000, Washington, DC 20004.

• HealthCare Abroad, 219 Investment Bldg., 1511 K St. N.W., Washington, DC 20005.

• American Association of Retired Persons. If you are a member, ask about the Medicare Supplement plan for travel. 1909 K St. N.W., Washington, DC 20049.

LOOKING AHEAD

All of this may sound like a lot to remember, but most travelers spend all of their time planning for a trip they may never enjoy — just because they have neglected to plan for their health needs.

Use the information sources at the end of this chapter, and the checklists, to help plan a happy journey.

IN SUMMARY:

— Carry enough prescription medicines to last for the whole trip.
— Visit your doctor and dentist, and take care of any medical problems before you leave.
— Pack medicines in hand-luggage that stays with you.
— Check your medical insurance to see whether it covers you abroad.

★ ★ ★
Travel Tool
★ ★ ★

TRAVELERS' HEALTH CLINICS

Here are some clinics specializing in pre-trip checkups, immunizations, and post-trip checkups — as well as telephone consultation to other physicians:

Mid-Atlantic — Traveler's Medical Service of Washington, 2141 K Street N.W., Washington, DC 20037 ☎ 202/466-8109.

Travelhealth Center, The Medical College of Pennsylvania, 3300 Henry Ave., Philadelphia, PA 19129 ☎ 215/842-6465.

Midwest — Travelers' Health Care Center, Division of Geographic Medicine, University Hospitals, Cleveland, OH 44106 ☎ 216/844-8081.

New England — Travelers' Health Service, New England Medical Center, 1750 Washington St., Boston, MA 02111; ☎ 617/956-7001.

271

New York — The International Health Care Service of The New York Hospital-Cornell Medical Center, 525 E. 68th St., New York NY 10021 ☎ 212/472-4284.

Northwest — University Hospital Travel and Medicine Service, University of Washington, Seattle, WA 98195 ☎ 206/548-4888.

South — Tropical Medicine and Travelers' Clinic, University of Miami Medical School, 1550 N.W. 10th Ave., Miami, FL 33125 ☎ 305/325-9845.

Travelers Health Clinic, Department of Tropical Medicine, Tulane Medical Center, 1501 Canal St., New Orleans, LA 70112 ☎ 504/588-5199.

Travelers Clinic, Division of Geographic Medicine, School of Medicine, Box 485, University of Virginia, Charlottesville, VA 22908 ☎ 804/924-9677.

Travel Well, a clinic operated by Emory University School of Medicine, Crawford Long Hospital of Emory University, 20 Linden Ave., Atlanta, GA 30365 ☎ 404/892-4411.

West Coast — Traveler's Clinic, UCSD Medical Center, 225 Dickinson St., San Diego, CA 92103 ☎ 619/543-2165.

★ ★ ★
Travel Tool
★ ★ ★

HEALTH ORGANIZATIONS

Here are some organizations that can help make your trip a healthier one:

• Citizens Emergency Center, Office of Consular Affairs, U.S. State Department, Washington, DC 20520 ☎ 202/632-5225. Offers various publications calling attention to health problems in different parts of the world.

• Immunization Alert, P.O. Box 406, Storrs, CT 06268 ☎ 203/487-0422. Personalized health information for travelers. Comprehensive reports include detailed advice on preventive shots and medications for travel in any country. Fee is $40 for a report covering up to four countries, $10 for each additional country.

• Intermedic, Inc., 777 Third Ave., New York, NY 10017 ☎ 212/486-8900. Worldwide network of English-speaking physicians who respond to emergency calls from its members. Personal membership costs $6 per year; family membership, $10.

• International Association for Medical Assistance to Travelers, 417 Center St., Lewiston, NY 14092 ☎ 716/754-4883. Nonprofit foundation to provide medical assistance to travelers in distress. Offers directory listing English-speaking doctors. Also publishes a *World Malaria Risk Chart*. Free membership.

• Worldwide Health Forecast Hotline ☎ 800/368-3531. Provided by HealthCare Abroad, an insurance company, the information available at this number is gathered from the Centers for Disease Control, the World Health Organization and the U.S. State Department. It is updated weekly or more often and describes health conditions in specific areas.

Travel Tool
★ ★ ★

READ MORE ABOUT IT

The health-conscious traveler can get more information from these sources:

Access Travel: Airports. A guide to accessibility of terminals. Write the U.S. Department of Health and Human Services, Washington, DC 20201. Free.

The Diabetic Traveler. Quarterly newsletter published by *The Diabetic Traveler*, P.O. Box 8223 RW, Stamford, CT 06905. Free.

Guide to International Dialysis. Type of dialysis offered at each center of the National Association of Patients on Hemodialysis and Transplantation, 150 Nassau St., New York, NY 10038 ☎ 212/619-2727. Free.

Health Information for International Travel (publication CDC 80-8280), published by the Centers for Disease Control. Send $4.75 to the Superintendent of Documents, U.S. Government Printing Office, Washington, D.C. 20402 ☎ 202/783-3238.

Tips for Travelers. A series of leaflets for each foreign country. Superintendent of Documents, Government Printing Office, Washington, DC 20402. $1.

Travel Tips for Senior Citizens. Superintendent of Documents, Government Printing Office, Washington, DC 20402. $1.

Your Trip Abroad. 32-page booklet, Superintendent of Documents, Government Printing Office, Washington, DC 20402. $1.

For those in need of even more help when traveling, try these books:

Access to the World, A Travel Guide for the Handicapped, by Louise Weiss, 1986. Published by Henry Holt and Company, New York.

The Physically Disabled Traveler's Guide, by Rod W. Durgin and Norene Lindsay, 1986. Published by Resource Directories, Toledo, Ohio.

Traveling Like Everybody Else, a practical guide for disabled travelers by Jacqueline Freedman and Susan Gersten, 1987. Published by Adama Books, New York.

★ ★ ★
Travel Tool
★ ★ ★

FOREIGN NAMES FOR COMMON NON-PRESCRIPTION DRUGS

Here are foreign brand names of some commonly used U.S. drugs. If the medicine you're taking isn't listed, ask your pharmacist for the generic name or the brand name it's sold under where you're going:

U.S. Drug	Used For	Generic Name	Foreign Brand
Actifed	Common cold	Pseudoephedrine w / triprolidine	Actifed, Linctifed
Aldactazide	Diuretic	Hydrochlorthiazide + spironolactone	Aldactide
Aldomet	High blood pressure	Methyldopa	Presinol (Belgium); Aldometil, Presinol, Sembrina (Germany); Aldomet, Medropren, Pesinol, Sembrina (Italy); Grospisk, Medopa, Methoplain (Japan)
Alupent	Asthma, breathing problems	Metaproterenol	Novasmasol (Italy);
Ativan	Tranquilizer, sleeping pill	Lorazepam	Tavor, Temestra (England); Control, Lorans, Quait, Securit (Italy); Wypax (Japan)
Butazolidin	Gout, arthritis, tendonitis, degenerative joint diseases	Phenylbutazone	Butacal, Butagesic, Butazolidin, Butazone Australia);Algoverine, Butagesic, Butazolidin, Intrabutazone, Malgesic, Nadozone Phenbutazone, Neo- zoline (Canada); Butazolidin Alka, Butacote, Butazone, Patrazolidin, Tibutazone (England); Butazolidine, Praecirheumin, Rheumapen, Spondyril, Mephabutazon, Ticinil Calcio (Germany); Butazolidine (France)

Brand Name	Use	Generic Name	Foreign Equivalents
Coumadin	Blood thinner	Warfarin	Warfilone, Warnerin (Canada); Coumadine (France, Germany, Italy, S. Africa) Algaphan (Australia)
Darvon	Pain reliever	Propoxyphene hydrochloride	Algodex, Depronal SA, Novaprogoxyn, Pro 65, 642 Tablets (Canada); Antivalc, Depronal(France); Evelin, Erantin (Germany); Lenigesial, Liberen, Tilene (Italy); Deprancol (Spain)
Glucotrol	Diabetes	Glipizide	Minodiab (Belgium, Denmark, England, France, Italy, Spain); Glipenese (Germany)
Isopto Carpine Eye Drops	Glaucoma	Pilocarpine	Adsorpocarpine, PV Carpine (Canada); Minims Pilocarpine Nitrate, Sno-pilo (England); Chibro-Pilocarpine, Dulcicarpine, Isopto Pilocarpine, Marticarpine, Pilo (France); Miopas, Pilocar, Piloman, Pilopos, Spersacarpin, Vistacarpine (Germany)
Isordil	Angina pectoris, heart pains	Isosorbide dinitrate	Carvasin, Isordil, Isotrate (Australia); Coronex, Isordil (Canada); Cedocard, Isoket Retard, Isordil, Isordil Tembids, Soni-slo, Sorbichew, Sorbide SA Sorbitrate, Vascardin (England); (France); Cardio, Corvliss, Isoket, Iso Mack, Maycor, Nitro, Nitrosorbon, Sorbidilat, Vermicet (Germany); Carvasin, Nitrosobide (Italy); Directran, Nitrol (Japan); Isorbid (Mexico)

Lomotil	Diarrhea, stomach cramps	Atropine Diphenoxylate	Retardin (Denmark, Norway, Sweden); Diarsed (France); Reasec (Italy)
Nitroglycerin	Angina pectoris, heart pains	Nitroglycerin	Anginine, Nitrolate, Sustac (Australia); Nitrol,Nitrong, Nitrostabilin, Nitrostat (Canada); Nitrocontin, Sustac (England); Lenitral (France); Gilucor Nitro, Klavikordal, Nitrangin, Nitrogesanit Retard Nitrolinguar, Nitro, Mack, Nitrorectal, Nitrozell-retard, Sustac-Retard, Trinitrosan (Germany); Lentronitrina, Nitroglyn, Nitrong, Nitro Retard, Venitrin (Italy)
Paraflex	Muscle relaxant	Chlorzoxazone	Biomioran (Italy); Escoflex (Switzerland)
Phenobartital	Sleeping pill, sedative	Phenobarbitol	Maliasin (Australia); Gardenal, Luminal, Nova-Pheno (Canada); Luminal, Parabal, Spansule, Phenobarbitone (England); Gardenal (France); Luminal, Luminaletten, Phenaemal, Phenaemaletten, Seda-Tablinen Germany); Luminal (Spain); Fenemal (Sweden)
Sudafed	Decongestant	Pseudophedrine	Drixora Repetabs, Sudelix (Australia); Eltor, Robidrine (Canada)

277

Tylenol	Fever reducer pain reliever	Acetaminophen	Bramcetamol, Calpon, Ceetamol, Dolamin, Dymadon, Pacemol, Panamax, Paracet, Parasin, Paraspen Parmol, Placemol, Tempra (Australia); Atasol, Campain, Exdol, Robigesic, Rounox, Tempra, Tivrin (Canada); Capol, Paldesic, Pamol, Panadol, Panasorb, Para-Seltzer, Ticelgesic, Unigesic (England); Doliprane (France); Anaflon, Ben-U-Ron (Germany); Acetamol, Nevral, Puernol, Tachipirina (Italy); Gelocatil, Melabon Infantil (Spain)
Valium	Muscle relaxer, Stress	Diazpam	Ducene, Lorinom, tranquilizer Propam (Australia); D-Tran, E-Pam, Meval, Neo-Calme, Novodipam, Paxel, Serenack, Pam, Vivol (Canada); Atensine, Diazemuls, Evacalm, Solis, Tensium, Valrelease (England); Euphorin, Sedaril, Sonacon (Japan)
Vibramycin	Antibiotic	Doxycycline	Vibramycin (Japan, Australia, England, France, Germany); Doxin (Australia); Vibraveinuse (France); Doxitard, Vibravenos (Germany); Hydramycin, Liomycin, Roximycin (Japan)

CHAPTER 21

PROTECTING YOURSELF

Being Prepared For It Can Head Off Trouble

A friend returning from Spain, a former marine who is 6' 2", told us how a group of small boys pinned his arms to his side in Madrid in broad daylight and stripped him of watch, rings and wallet while he watched helplessly. The same thing could have happened to him, of course, in his hometown of Philadelphia.

On the other hand, we have a petite woman friend who used her purse as a weapon to ward off a throng of Gypsy children in front of the Louvre. She simply took the purse by its handles and swung it around herself screaming bloody murder until help arrived. She didn't lose a thing.

Pickpockets and muggers operate around the world — including the town where you live. And when they strike, your only safeguards are your alertness and composure. Even using those diligently, you may not be able to prevent theft and robbery.

The only difference between keeping safe on the road and keeping safe at home is that traveling takes you into strange surroundings and not along familiar paths to your favorite park or department store. But while having fun on a trip, you may not keep your guard up as conscientiously as you would at home.

It is precisely the strangeness of a new place you're visiting — newness, if you will — that makes you act tentatively, sending the kind of signals would-be troublemakers are looking for.

When reading these suggestions to help you keep safe while traveling, you may think — Wow! That's too much to worry about. And decide to stay home. Don't. Get up and go and enjoy yourself. The truth is that very few travelers run into serious problems. But we believe that prevention is far and away the best safeguard against potential problems. So we do the best we can, using the safeguards that fit us, and keep on going and enjoying.

DOING YOUR HOMEWORK

Learn as much as you can about the places you'll be going to. Your travel agent's is a good place to start. Ask if your agent has been to the places you will be visiting and if so, ask the kinds of questions you would pose to a relative or friend who has just returned from a trip.

Ask about hotels and what kind of fire-safety precautions, such as sprinkler systems, are used. Ask whether any airports and airlines along your route have had security slip-ups. And, finally, ask your agent for literature and recommended reading sources.

Follow up by visiting your library or bookstore to locate recent books, magazine articles and videos about your destinations.

Get current maps of the cities where you'll be staying. Mark your hotel location on each city map. Ask questions about areas to avoid and mark those on the maps, too. Find out whether the streets around your hotel are considered safe for walking. Ask about nearby public transportation and whether it's considered safe to use. People who can supply such information about your hotel area and city include your travel agent, consulate office, tour guide, hotel security people, desk clerk and concierge.

Read your daily newspapers carefully, noting incidents occurring at and near your destinations. Or check *The New York Times* monthly index, which will list specific incidents of terrorism.

Learn words like "help," "police" and "fire" in the languages of the countries you'll be visiting. (Some of the words you need are at the end of this chapter).

Pay in advance for as many tours and services as possible, and carry vouchers for them when you travel, to limit the amount of money you have to carry.

Memorize your passport number so you don't need to take it out each time identification is needed.

Use the resources of your federal government. The U.S. Department of State (Bureau of Consular Affairs, Washington, DC 20524) issues travel advisories about countries throughout the world. They are free for the asking and describe situations ranging from special holidays to revolution, country by country. The Citizen's Emergency Center of the Bureau of Consular Affairs also maintains a telephone hotline, ☎ 202/647-5225, from 8:30 a.m. to 10 p.m. (EST) Monday through Friday for the latest information on safety conditions in any part of the world. The Superintendent of Documents (Government Printing Office, Washington DC 20502) supplies *Background Notes* about the countries you're planning to visit; just ask for them. And read them.

PACKING FOR SAFETY

Unwittingly, people send signals about what good targets they are for burglars and thieves. A person carrying leather designer luggage and wearing obviously expensive jewelry is wearing a billboard that reads, "Rob me, it's worth your while."

For that reason, plan your travel wardrobe so you'll fit into the crowd and avoid calling attention to yourself.

Choose well-made, inexpensive, lightweight luggage with sturdy locks. Remove all decals and labels that proclaim you as a world traveler or as an important person. Replace them with straight-forward identification using a business address (without a company name) — rather than a home address — if possible. Put duplicate identification inside each bag. Some travelers prefer to tag their luggage with the address of the hotel they're heading for; that way, if it's lost, the luggage will go to you and not away from you.

Choose a camera that is unobtrusive — preferably one small enough to fit into a pocket or purse.

Choose a device, such as a money belt or necklace-style billfold, to carry your money, credit cards, international driver's license, passport and visas. The purse and back pocket are the worst locations for these important papers. If you are traveling with a spouse, divide the money and cards between you.

Some travelers show enormous creativity. They carry valuables in a photographer's vest or a string-net shopping bag. They wrap billfolds in rubber bands to make them more difficult to remove. They'll sew Velcro fasteners to the sides of each pocket opening to help protect valuables.

Take along an extra passport photo — and keep it in a place separate from where you keep the passport. Then if your passport is stolen or lost, replacement will be quicker.

Take just one or two credit cards and only a few personal checks. To select the credit cards you want, determine which additional services the card company offers that you believe will be useful (cash advances, travel insurance, convenient ATMs) and ask the company how widely their card is accepted in the places you plan to visit.

And make a list of check numbers, along with credit-card numbers, your passport number, ticket number and emergency telephone numbers (your travel agent, where to report lost credit cards and passports, your physician and so on). Keep these numbers with your duplicate prescriptions for medicine and eyeglasses.

Take only costume jewelry. Avoid jewelry that indicates you're an important person, such as membership pins or other insignia.

Clean out your billfold and remove things that proclaim your value, such as country-club membership cards or armed forces identification. If you are required to carry your military ID, keep it where it can be easily hidden.

Women should choose a purse that provides maximum protection against theft. For example, a leather bag will not be as easy as a fabric one for a thief to cut away from its handles or cut across the bottom to allow the contents to fall out. A shoulder-strap bag has handles long enough to allow you to wear it across your chest or to wrap the handle around your wrist. And choose a purse with a zipper top and one or two zipper pockets inside.

Use common sense when packing your carry-on bag. It may have to be opened by airport security people, so valuables should not be laid loosely and temptingly on top.

Lock your luggage after it is packed.

PREPARING FOR DEPARTURE

The hustle and bustle of an airport, depot or dock is the ideal spot to lose touch with your possessions and tickets. In fact, law-enforcement officials often call such places a crime zone because the thieves have found the pickings so lush. Keep alert to your surroundings and keep an eagle eye on your luggage, and you're likely to be more secure.

Leave home with adequate time to allow for the unknown and unexpected, such as an accident delaying traffic. When you're rushed, you're less likely to notice things that can put you in jeopardy.

If your journey is a short one, you'll probably drive your own car and leave it. Choose a well-lighted area of the parking lot or garage. Lock your car securely and take your parking ticket with you; don't leave it in the car, where a thief can make use of it.

If your journey is a longer one, you may be relying on cabs or shuttles to get you to your departure point. If so, start practicing the hardest and most effective safety lesson of all — keeping your mouth shut. Be discreet. No one — cab driver or shuttle companion — needs to know where you're going or how long you'll be gone.

If your journey is a very long one, the amount of luggage, alone, provides helpful information to thieves; you might want to drive your luggage to your departure point the day before you're scheduled to leave and put it in a locker. Then you can use public transportation — cabs, buses or shuttles — safely on your departure day. No one will suspect you're leaving town if you're not carrying luggage.

If you need friends or neighbors to take you, try to choose the same people that will be looking out for your home. That way, you limit the number of people who will know you're out of town.

Keep an eye on your luggage at all times. You'll avoid being the victim of such scams as "the catsup man," a person who squirts catsup on your back. (While you're busy trying to see and remove the stain, your luggage heads out the door.)

When you arrive, check your luggage and verify that the tags put on it match your destination. Move through the security checkpoints and into the security areas as quickly as possible.

Maintain a low profile by talking quietly, by keeping your patience when standing in lines and by not creating scenes.

Choose an airplane seat away from exits, away from the front of the plane, away from bathrooms and away from the aisles, all areas that terrorists have need to control.

When your airplane tickets are returned to you, make sure only the necessary tickets were removed and that you have all the tickets you need remaining for the trip.

When going through security, avoid disputes.

Say no if people you don't know well ask you to carry packages or envelopes for them. If you see unattended luggage, report it to officials.

When conducting pick-up conversations in airports, depots or docks, avoid volunteering information that could be helpful to dishonest people or terrorists. As Jack Adler and Thomas C. Tompkins suggest in their book, *Travel Safety*, " ... try listening to a nearby conversation while at an airport. See how much you can piece together about the people doing the talking. You might be amazed ... "

PREPARING FOR ARRIVAL

Arriving at a strange place can cause you to be distracted and thus an easier mark than you would normally be. Be attentive when disembarking from your plane, train or ship. Notice where exits are, where the luggage collection points are and where ground transportation is located. Basically, it's a matter of getting your bearings so you can move with determination.

If you're jostled, turn quickly — you may avoid being a pickpocket's victim. By the same token, avoid having your attention diverted by any means — it can be a ploy to set you up as a victim. The usual pickpocket's diversions are created by one person so a second person can steal your valuables. They can include a lovers' quarrel, bands of roaming, begging children, loud noises, a request for you to take someone's photo or a "lost" person. But they all have the same goal: to force you to drop your guard.

If you take a cab to your hotel, avoid those vehicles that appear to be one of a kind — sometimes called "Gypsy" cabs or independents. Also check to make sure the driver's photo matches the person behind the wheel. If the driver has a companion, choose a different vehicle. Ignore a driver who tells you your hotel is full or closed; it may be a ploy to earn a commission by taking you to another hotel.

If you rent a car at your destination, choose a modest one that allows you a way to store your luggage out of sight of prying eyes. Avoid leaving maps and guidebooks in plain sight; they reveal that the car is driven by a stranger to the area. Refuse cars that carry United States decals or tourist identification.

Keep your rental car papers with your passport and other important documents.

Thoroughly check out the car before you start driving it. Make sure everything is in good working condition — brakes, lights, locks, air conditioning, tires and the like.

When you drive a rented vehicle, stay on well-traveled and well-lighted roads. Keep valuables, such as purses, on the floor, and lock the car doors. When you park, choose areas protected by your hotel or business or a well-lighted street. One very savvy traveler always chooses highway exits marked by hospital signs (the blue circle with the white "H" in the middle) when traveling alone at night. As he points out, a hospital operates 24 hours, is well-lighted with people in and around it, and it has telephones and food — exactly the things he's likely to need at night.

Some tourists have been accosted while dealing with a disabled car. If your car conks out, head for a service station, or stay in the locked car with emergency lights flashing. If you have a flat tire, only one person should get out to look or attempt to change the tire. The second person should stay inside the locked car with windows rolled up. A flat tire can be a thief's diversionary tactic to get you to stop.

If you choose public transportation, ask the hotel personnel such as the desk clerk or concierge what kind of areas it travels through going to your destination so you won't put yourself in jeopardy. Ask about special, local holidays that could interfere with normal traffic and learn the hours the buses run so you won't strand yourself. Choose a seat near the driver. If carrying a purse, don't set it unattended on your lap or the floor. Keep it close to your body with the handle wrapped around your wrist.

If you're walking, choose the center portion of the sidewalk — away from the curb side where motorcycle bandits ply their trade. Just as you would at home, avoid dark, deserted streets and alleyways.

Carry a noisemaker, like a referee's whistle, to call for help if it's needed.

Carry as little money with you as possible.

Keep a matchbook, card or some other printed material with your hotel's name, address and phone number on it as well as identification with your own name and address. If your walk takes you shopping, take these precautions:

• Make sure your credit card is returned after your transaction, and destroy the carbons.

• Keep the copy of your credit-card charge slips or itemized receipts in case you want to return the item or to use for customs.

• Avoid displaying large amounts of cash or great numbers of credit cards.

• Check your change.

• Thumb through your traveler's checks periodically to verify the number sequence. Sometimes thieves will take a check or two from the center of the pack, duplicate your signature and cash them.

• Mail small purchases home, and be particularly alert when transporting your purchases back to your hotel.

CHECKING OUT YOUR ROOM

Checking into your hotel should be simple, but there are things that will help make it safer, too. For a start, don't turn over your bags or your car to a porter or bellhop who's out of uniform.

To prevent the clerk from announcing your name, room number or length of stay — all important information for working thieves — just say you have a reservation and present your credit card.

Ask about the hotel safe, and use it for your valuables. Be sure to get a receipt for them.

Always request a room on floors three through six and away from the street. They're considered safest because lower floors are easier targets for break-ins, and higher floors are more difficult for fire-fighting equipment to reach.

You should be taken to your room by hotel personnel. Your escort should unlock and enter your room first, turning on lights and checking to see that things work. You need to make sure there are working fire detectors and working locks on windows or sliding doors and on the doors with access to another room. Also verify that the locks on the main doors are adequate and working; if not, ask for a different room.

HOTEL SAFETY

Most hotels and motels in the United States are fire-resistant, and many older ones were shut down or forced to modernize after the fatal fires at the Las Vegas MGM Grand and the DuPont Plaza in San Juan, Puerto Rico. Hotels overseas, however, may not be as safe.

At most U.S. inns, rooms are fitted with smoke detectors and sprinklers. Escape routes are posted on the backs of room doors. In some places, bellhops and other hotel employees are trained in fire safety — how to notify guests, how to prevent panic, how to stop a fire from spreading and the like — and are encouraged to talk about it with guests.

Right after you get settled in to your room, make these steps a required ritual — a fire check at a hotel is just as important as a lifeboat drill on a cruiseship:

• Walk the halls to the emergency exits, counting doorways and noting other landmarks like ice machines. Some experts recommend that you draw a map and keep it with your hotel key on the night-table to avoid confusion during an emergency. And remember, never count on using the elevator in a fire.

• Find the fire extinguishers on your floor and memorize their locations.

• Make sure your windows open, and figure out how the latches work.

• Look outside to see whether the window offers another practical fire escape.

Have your room key within reach when you go to sleep, so you can find it even in the dark. And if fire breaks out, take the key with you — if you can't get through the hallway, you may have to return to your room.

Few people are actually burned to death in hotel fires. Most die from smoke, poison gases and panic.

Should fire break out in your room, don't try to control it —
call the operator right away, leave the room and close the door
behind you, and begin knocking on doors to arouse your neighbors. If fire breaks out elsewhere in the hotel, grab your key and
head for the door; if you smell gases or smoke in your room, roll
out of bed onto the floor and find the door. If the door handle is
hot, don't open it — that means there's fire in the hallway.

If there's already smoke in your room, open your window to
vent it — break the window, if you have to. Now's the time to
jump if you're below the fourth floor — most people survive
jumps of 35 feet or less. If heat and flames are rising outside the
window from a lower floor, don't breathe smoke-laden air.

Turn on the bathroom fan to help clear the smoke; fill the
bathtub with water. Wet down towels and sheets and stuff them
around doors or any other crack where smoke is seeping in. Use
a blanket to make a tent over your head and sit at the open
window to get fresh air.

If you're forced to leave your room as a last resort, remember
to keep low.

If your fire detector goes off, contact the hotel desk immediately and ask for instructions.

There are now many kinds of keys for hotel rooms — from
the old-fashioned variety to plastic cards to a personal identification number input into a computer. There are legitimate
differences of opinion about whether to leave your key with the
desk clerk or to take it with you each time you leave the hotel. A
compromise is to leave it with the desk when heading for the
beach or tennis courts — places where light-fingered types
would be able to pick up your key from under your towel or
shoe. And take it along the rest of the time. In any case, never
display your room key in public.

When you leave your room, turn the radio or television on
low volume and don't use the sign that tells the hotel staff to
make up the room; it also tells thieves you're not there. Avoid
leaving important or expensive items in your room.

While in your room, keep your door locked and don't open
it to any unexpected people — even those claiming to be hotel
personnel. If you don't know them or why they are there, take a
moment to call the front desk and ask before unlocking your

door. Keep luggage and other impediments out of the path to the front door.

You may want to do just the opposite in a train's sleeping car. A piece of luggage in front of the door may be just the right deterrent to keep a thief from slipping into your compartment.

When traveling by train or motorcoach, daytime travelers can doze off to become a pickpocket's target, and those traveling overnight will need to hide their valuables while they sleep. Many travelers wear their money belts or pouches to bed; some use their purses as pillows.

PREPARING FOR THE WORST

Being in the wrong place at the wrong time often has more to do with whether you become enmeshed in terrorism, but much of the anti-terrorist advice given to Americans you've already read in this chapter:

• Blend with the local crowds.

• Don't volunteer information about yourself or family.

• Don't identify yourself as a person of wealth, importance or with the military.

• Stay alert.

If you want to find out more about personal security, here are some things you can read:

Countering Terrorism, Department of State Publication 8884. Write Consumer Information Center, Pueblo, CO 81004.

The Pocket Guide to Safe Travel by Dr. Stephen Sloan, a specialist in terrorism. $3.25. Contemporary Books, Inc., 180 N. Michigan Ave., Chicago, IL 60601.

Travel Safety: Safe Guards at Home and Abroad by Jack Adler and Thomas C. Tompkins. $14.95. Hippocrene Books, 171 Madison Ave., New York NY 10016.

IN SUMMARY

— Learn as much as you can about where you're going
— Keep a low profile
— Keep alert
— Be unpredictable

Travel Tool
★ ★ ★

WHAT TO YELL WHEN YOU'RE IN TROUBLE

Here are some foreign phrases which can help you overseas. Don't be afraid to yell when you're in trouble:

French
Fire: Au feu (oa fur)
Help: Au secours (oa serkoor)
Police: Police (polesss)
Get a doctor: Appelez un médecin (ah-perlay ang maydssang)

German
Fire: Feuer (foyerr)
Help: Hilfe (hilfer)
Police: Polizei (politsigh)
Get a doctor: Holen sie einen Arzt (hoalern zee ighnern ahrtst)

Spanish
Fire: Fuego (fway oa)
Help: Socorro (sokoarroa)
Police: Policía (poaleetheeash)
Get a doctor: Busque un doctor (booskay oon doaktor)

Italian
Fire: Al fuoco (ahi fwawkoa)
Help: Aiuto (aheeootoa)
Police: Polizia (poaleetseeah)
Get a doctor: Chiami un medico (keeaamee oon maideekoa)

Portuguese
Fire: Fogo (foagoo)
Help: Socorro (sookoarroo)
Police: Policia (pooleessyer)
Get a doctor: Chame urn medico (shermer oong mehdikkoo)

Japanese
Fire: Kaji
Help: Tasukete
Police: Keisatsu
Get a doctor: Isha o yonde kudasai

Russian
Fire: Pahzhahr
Help: Nah pomahshch
Police: Meelyeetsiyah
Get a doctor: Pahzahveetyee vrah-chyah

Polish
Fire: Pozhahr
Help Rahtoonkoo
Police: Meeleets-yah
Get a doctor: Prosheh vehzvahtsh leh-kahzhah)

Swedish
Fire: Elden ar los (ehldern aer lurss)
Help: Hjälp (yehlp)
Police: Polis (poleess)
Get a doctor: Hamta en läkare (hehmtah ehn laikahrer)

Foreign terminology is provided courtesy of Berlitz Language Centers.

CHAPTER 22

HELP!

> If You're In Trouble Abroad, Make the Consulate
> Your First Friend

An American couple, just arrived in Munich on a group tour, sets out on foot to explore the town. Late in the day they realize they don't know the name of their new hotel, and can't possibly find their way back to it, since they can't speak the language.

An American youth, dirty and broke, wanders with his guitar into the U.S. Embassy in London, trying to find out how to sell a kidney to raise funds to get home.

The U.S. Consulate comes to the rescue!

The Munich visitors see the U.S. consular officer, who calls 20 hotels before finding the couple's name on a register and then directs them back to their group.

The U.S. consular officer in London can't give medical aid to the youth, since there isn't any medical emergency. But he can help the lad wire home for money to pay his airfare out of England.

It's all in a day's work for U.S. consular officers in 250 embassies and other offices throughout the world. Helping strangers in a strange land with a strange language is their job. If you are in trouble overseas, make the consulate your first friend.

WHAT THE CONSULATE CAN (AND CAN'T) DO

While you may be entitled to full protection of the Constitution inside an American embassy, you have to conduct yourself according to local laws and cope with local customs when you're traveling abroad.

Though it happens rarely, you could even be jailed for some inadvertent action that you think is innocent. You could have a bottle of schnapps in your bag when you're trying to enter some Moslem country; you could be caught with a narcotic medicine you forgot to bring a prescription for; you could be arrested for taking a photo of the wrong military installation on a visit behind the Iron Curtain.

More usual emergencies are losing your money or passport, becoming ill or having a traveling companion die. The consular officer is the one charged with helping you should any of those calamities occur.

Here are some typical things an American consular officer can do:

• Issue a replacement passport if yours is lost or stolen.

• Help find missing Americans.

• Help you find medical assistance, including English-speaking doctors, and inform your relatives at home that there's an emergency.

• If you're out of money, help you get emergency cash wired from home or your bank (and even lend you up to $50 to tide you over until the emergency cash arrives).

• Help you find legal assistance if you're arrested, and help you get funds from home to post bail.

• Watch over you in jail, try to relieve any unsafe or unhealthy conditions there, provide supplementary diet items and notify your relatives.

• Provide notary and witnessing services.

• Help you cast an absentee ballot.

• In the event of a death overseas, help with the paperwork and shipping the body home.

• In the event of civil unrest or a natural disaster, help protect you and get you out of the country.

The consular officer can't pay your medical or legal bills, put up bail, settle disputes with hotels or local merchants, act as interpreter, search for missing luggage or do any other work of a travel agent, an information booth or a bank.

Basically, the consulate is there to help with your emergencies. If you've been robbed in Rotterdam or had your pocket picked in Paris, the consular officer can advise you what to do to get your trip back on track.

If you're visiting a sensitive area, it's a good idea to check in with the consular officer with a copy of your itinerary as soon as you arrive, so he knows you're there and where to get in touch. If you're on an escorted tour, the guide will take care of that for you.

BEFORE YOU LEAVE HOME

Of course, if you can't find a consular office, you can't get help there.

Before you leave home, write down the numbers of U.S. consulates in the countries you'll be visiting. For a list of them, send $4.25 for the booklet *Key Officers of Foreign Service Posts* to Superintendent of Documents, U.S. Government Printing Office, Washington, DC 20402. Keep the phone numbers and addresses in several different places — in your wallet, in your luggage, with your companion.

Call the Department of State's Citizen's Emergency Center at ☎ 202/647-5225 to check on what is happening in the places you plan to visit — advisories are put out on things like uprisings, floods, disease, restrictions on travel, nuclear fallout and other calamities you want to avoid.

And make out a detailed itinerary, including dates, lodgings and phone numbers where you'll be staying, to leave behind with relatives or friends.

That will make it easier to trace you, if needed.

THE CITIZEN'S EMERGENCY CENTER

As well as an information source, the Citizen's Emergency Center can also be the hotline for friends or relatives who need to contact you while you're traveling. They can use the center to help:
- Get information if you've been arrested.
- Find you, if you're not where you're supposed to be.
- Transmit money to you in an emergency.
- Arrange medical evacuation if you get sick.

The center is normally open weekdays from 8:15 a.m. to 10 p.m. (EST). But if there's a real emergency after hours, you can get help by calling ☎ 202/634-3600 and asking for the Overseas Citizen's Services (OCS) duty officer.

OTHER OVERSEAS HELPERS

More complete help than a consulate can give you is available through companies like Travel Assistance International (TAI) or Access America.

Basically an insurance company, TAI, for example, gives you a local number to call in an overseas emergency for all kinds of help. Unlike the consulate, TAI will pay your medical bills, bail you out of jail, give you emergency cash, pay for your ticket home or pay to fly a relative to your bedside.

Even considering that it includes trip insurance, lost-baggage insurance and short-term health insurance, the cost isn't cheap: $40 a person for a week of travel, or $120 for a year's protection. But the peace of mind, especially if you're visiting a Third-World country, probably is worth it.

You can join TAI or other such groups through your travel agent or your credit-card company, or contact directly: Travel Assistance International, 1133 15th St. N.W., Washington, DC 20005 ☎ (800/821-2828). For a listing of other similar organizations, see Chapter 20, To Your Health.

Here are other ways to get help overseas:

If your car breaks down — If you're an AAA member, you can get free road services, towing or other maintenance from affiliated foreign auto clubs just by phoning, as you would in America (see Chapter 10, By Automobile). To get the phone numbers, ask your local AAA office for the booklet *Offices To Serve You Abroad*.

If you lose your credit card — Phone the nearest credit-card office. American Express claims it can reissue another card within 24 hours. In addition, if you don't have your card number, they'll find it on their computer. Other credit cards can take longer — Diner's Club up to two days and some bank cards up to two weeks. They'll give you local numbers to phone to report lost cards.

If you lose your traveler's checks — Immediately phone the company that issued them. If you've kept the numbers, you can usually get replacement checks the same day. When you buy your checks, find out what numbers to call and what the replacement procedure is.

Other emergencies — There's no record of your hotel reservations or your flight. You want to change your schedule. You've gotten on the wrong train. And so on. Especially if you don't speak the language, your travel agent should provide you with the name of a colleague in the country you're visiting to sort out things like that.

BE PREPARED

You can't use all the emergency services available to you unless you do some advance preparation:

• Make lists: your passport number, credit-card numbers, traveler's-check numbers (along with amounts and the issuer's name), airline-ticket numbers. Keep the lists separate from the original documents. Have your traveling companion carry duplicate lists.

• Make several copies of your itinerary. Give one to a friend at home, tape one inside your luggage (so if it's lost, whoever finds it can catch up with you), keep one, have several extras for the consulate.

• Have extra passport photos and proof of your American citizenship.

• Write down phone numbers: airline, your hotel, traveler's-check and credit-card replacement numbers, home numbers of family and friends, numbers of U.S. consulates where you're visiting, auto club, emergency-insurance company, your travel agent (or his colleague).

IN SUMMARY:

— If you have a medical or legal emergency, or lose your passport or money, contact a U.S. consular officer.
— If you're visiting a sensitive area, check in with the consular officer right away.
— Some private companies and organizations also can help in emergencies.

NOTES

IV

PLACES

Here are some places that seniors favor, and some places that favor seniors.

CHAPTER 23

TRAVELS FOR 49ERS-PLUS

> There's No Such Thing as a Best Place for Seniors

There is no doubt about mature travelers' favorite ways to travel:

Cruiseship, RV, motorcoach.

There's plenty of research to support that.

But ask any tour industry expert or researcher about mature travelers' favorite places, and there's silence. The truth is, there's no such thing as a favored place for mature travelers. We like the same places that other age-groups favor. Sure, cruising to Alaska, is clearly one of our favorite trips. Golly, it's a great trip for anyone, whether 22 or 82. Same for Hawaii.

The authors like Venice; many mature travelers hate it. You have to walk everywhere — vehicles aren't permitted. The streets are narrow, the crowds thick, the pigeons intrusive, many of the shops tacky. But we're walkers, gallery-goers, photographers — and Venice is great for us.

We like Burgundy, and we visit the California wine country frequently. But if you don't care much about wine, you'd probably be bored in Beaune, France, or Napa, Calif., whatever your age. So we recommend those places for those who appreciate wine, not necessarily for mature travelers.

Florida's not our favorite place — too flat, among other things, and too hot some months. But mature travelers flock to Florida by the millions. Just our taste — no reflection on Florida. Shucks, we don't even like Paris very much.

The truth is that the best places to visit depends entirely on your own tastes and budget — not how old you are.

BEST PLACES FOR SENIORS

Once we tried to compile a list of seniors' favorite places. "The national parks," said one tour packager. "Our older customers most often take the national parks trip." Of course, her motorcoach tours didn't go east of the Mississippi, so how could she name Washington, or Florida? "The seniors' favorite is the Costa del Sol," said a spokesman from Saga Holidays, which is a very large tour operator for mature travelers and can pull such statistics out of its computers — an authority on senior travel. But Saga rarely runs tours to Alaska or Texas, so how would they know?

We asked others with the same result. All the places named were great for seniors to visit, and for lots of other people, too. But we don't believe anyone has ever discovered the 10 or 12 "best senior destinations." We don't even believe it's possible to come up with a list like that.

The usually reliable Prentice Hall *Places Rated* books offer no clues, either. *Vacation Places Rated* gives you some good ideas of where to go, but it evaluates only domestic places — not low-cost Mexico or lovely Canada. *Retirement Places Rated* is great if you're going to retire — but you're not going to spend a gala two-week vacation in Iowa City, Iowa, or Murray, Ky. (some recent favorites), no matter how great the medical facilities and the bus systems are.

VACATION PLACES RATED (AND UNRATED)

There's no doubt that tourism figures show Alaska, Hawaii and Mexico to be favorite destinations for U.S. and Canadian seniors. After that, as we said, other favorites are anybody's guess. Even so, we want to try our hand at a list, based on talk we've heard over the years. Call it Our Travel Insiders' Dozen Great Places for 49ers-Plus. Simply, they're places we think will be your favorites:

Alaska — Nowhere else can you see icebergs being formed as you watch. And the ride on the deluxe McKinley Explorer through Denali National Park is one of the world's choice train rides.

Alaska, at its best, is a cruise experience. You'll leave from Vancouver, cruise the Inside Passage to Juneau, Glacier Bay and Skagway, then on to Anchorage. Take the train from there through Denali, with an overnight stopover at a lodge in the park, to Fairbanks; fly back to Anchorage, then back to Seattle. Or work it in the other direction: Fly up and cruise back.

There are sidetrips on the Yukon Queen riverboat, the White Pass & Yukon narrow-gauge railroad from Whitehorse to Skagway and the cruiseship Ptarmigan for a close-in look at Portage Glacier.

Along the way, you'll get your fill of glaciers and migrating whales, a look at what the West might have been like today if it had stayed the West, along with all the joys of ocean cruising. Lots of cruiselines make the Alaska run. One, World Explorer, even features scholarly lectures on things like geology and Alaska history as you sail.

A popular trip for RVers in the summer is the Alaska Marine Highway, a ferry system plying the Inside Passage that serves the state's coastal communities. Pick up the ferry at Seattle, or drive up to Prince Rupert, B.C. You can drive your rig right onto the boat, spend overnight in a private cabin, cruise to the first town, get off and go camping. Then you can get back on the ferry with your RV and visit the next town. Using the low-cost ferry, you can spend a whole summer camping along Alaska southern coast, all the way out to the Aleutians. From October to May, you can travel free if you're over 65 (you still pay for your vehicle).

For schedules and fares, write Alaska Marine Highway, P.O. Box R, Juneau, AK 99811 (toll-free 800/642-0066).

Hawaii — Tourism is Hawaii's biggest business, and one-third of the mainland visitors to Hawaii are 49ers-plus: more than 1.2 million of us each year. And we stay longer—an average of 12 nights, compared with the average visit of seven nights.

No wonder — savvy seniors have discovered the lovely outer islands — Molokai, Kauai, Maui and the towering Big Island, Hawaii. Only 52 percent of travelers over 49 spend the whole visit in teeming Honolulu — the average for other age groups is 78 percent. More than half of all visitors to the shopping island of Maui and tiny Kauai, the garden island, are 49ers-plus.

Visitors who limit themselves to Honolulu don't know that most of Hawaii is rural — but rural means something else there: lava fields instead of prairies, rain forests instead of piney woods, sugar-cane fields instead of wheat fields.

While surfing may lure the youngsters, we are particularly fetched by the culture of the islands, and the stories of how they came to be: how the demigod Maui climbed Mt. Haleakala to harness the sun, how the little people called Menehunes built and still guard the island of Kauai, how fiery Pele of the volcanoes continues to rule the landscape and the lives of the people of the Big Island.

Not to be missed are the Arizona Monument at Pearl Harbor, the Polynesian Culture Center, Iolani Palace and the Bishop Museum on Oahu; deep, colorful Waimea Canyon on Kauai; the volcano show on Hawaii, the Big Island; and Whaler's Village at Kaanapali, the drive to Hana and the visit to the Haleakala crater on Maui.

You can buy tour packages that will fly you from island to island, but we think the best way to see Hawaii is aboard ship — American-Hawaii Cruises' SS Constitution or SS Independence. You'll get two- or three-day Honolulu visits before or after your week cruising the outer islands. The cost ranges from $1,000 to $3,500, including airfare. There are also fly/cruise combinations, if you don't have time for a longer visit.

But why would you want to hurry home from this haunting place? While Alaska seems to be many seniors' No. 1 destination, Hawaii is ours.

Mexico — Mexico has almost everything a mature traveler could want. There is lots to see, costs are low, the climate inland is moderate, and the people seem to like to have you there. Don't worry about the language. Most service people and shopkeepers in the tourist areas speak English. Menus are in English and sometimes German, as well as Mexican.

Favorite destinations for seniors are Guadalajara and Lake Chapala, where there are big American retirement communities. It's a good trip for summer as well as winter months. So is the drive from Mexico City to Cuernavaca. RV caravans into Mexico, mounted out of Texas and New Mexico, are also popular. A trip gaining popularity is the rail trip through Copper Canyon, from

Chihuahua to Los Mochis on the Gulf of California (see Chapter 14, By Rail), plus a ferry ride over to La Paz in Baja California.

For winter breaks, anywhere along the west coast from Acapulco to Mazatlán is comfortable, and so are the prices, even for high season. From Cancún on the Caribbean side you can explore old ruins, as well as take in the sunshine. And sleepy Loreto on the Baja coast, a Humphrey Bogart kind of village now, is likely to be the hot destination of the 1990s. It's under development by Fonatur (an agency of the Mexican government), just as Zihuatanejo, another sleepy Humphrey Bogart kind of town, was under development for the '80s. That became the popular resort of Ixtapa.

A budget tip: for even lower prices, visit Mexico's coastal areas in the shoulder months of April-May and October-November. It's warm, but tolerable, and only moderately rainy. Ask your travel agent exactly when the prices change.

Africa — East Africa is one of the most exciting places left in the world to visit. Some tour operators put together African packages particularly attractive to mature travelers.

When we were kids, we read all about Africa in the Martin and Osa Johnson books — now we can see places like Mombasa, Kenya and its capital, Nairobi, and Mount Kilimanjaro for ourselves. We can see the seas of animals Martin Johnson saw, and film the natives Martin Johnson filmed.

Though it's on the Equator, the climate is uncomfortable only along the seacoast. On the inland highlands — which is most of the country — one writer describes it as "much like the Rio Grand Valley in New Mexico," with a dry heat during the day and cool evenings. Inland Nairobi is typically 10 to 15 degrees cooler than Mombasa, on the seacoast, and Nairobi's spring rainy season lasts only half as long as Mombasa's. If you have respiratory problems, check with your doctor before you book a trip. There's lots of dust on the animal preserves. Take the usual health precautions you would for any Third-World country.

Don't try to do East Africa on your own — take a package tour. Typically, they range from 12 to 21 days and cost $3,500-$5,000, including airfare from U.S. gateways. Don't book a tour that puts you in the cities for any length of time — you visit Africa to get out into the bush and see the animals. By day, you'll roam the game preserves in a four-wheel-drive Land Rover; at night you'll stay at a unique game lodge like The Ark or Treetops, where the animals wander up close, or in a tented camp, as in the old days of safari. Make sure your itinerary includes the Masai Mara National Reserve, Samburu National Reserve and Amboseli National Park.

Hemphill Harris has some particularly thorough tours; some include gorilla tracking in nearby Rwanda. Saga Holidays also has some good East Africa packages exclusively for seniors at around $3,500. One packager, African Travel, recently offered travelers over 55 a 16-day safari for the price of 14 days — $3,800 — plus an extra free week in South Africa for seniors booking 16- and 20-day safaris.

Canadian Rockies/Vancouver — To some, Vancouver is a lot like San Francisco, though less expensive — and less frantic, too. There are flowers everywhere. Homes are covered with them; they hang from the lightpoles; they're in every open space in public places. It seems as if you can't get away from the flowers — Vancouver is like a giant garden. And clean. Moreover, there's lots to see and do nearby: the Canadian Rockies, quaint Victoria and Seattle, all less than a day's journey.

The best time to visit Vancouver is in the summer — mid-June to mid-September. Days are bright and crisp, with highs in the upper 70s and little rain. Otherwise, like San Francisco, it gets chilly and rainy — even foggy.

On the other hand, if you're arriving by train, the snowy Canadian Rockies, always beautiful, are at their best in the winter.

Prices are right for mature travelers in Canada. You won't get sticker shock, even when prices are quoted in Canadian dollars. Most hotels offer the usual senior-citizen rates. And Air Canada has deep discounts — up to 50 percent — for travelers 65 or older from U.S. cities.

But Vancouver should be a train trip — and both Via Rail Canada and Amtrak have deep discounts for mature travelers. Take the Amtrak's Empire Builder from Chicago or the Upper Midwest, through the Cascades to Seattle. Or the spectacular Coast Starlight run up from Los Angeles and San Francisco. Spend a few days in Seattle, then take the ferry to Vancouver, stopping off to see Victoria, even more of a flowered city than Vancouver. After your Vancouver stay, climb aboard Via Rail for a breathtaking run through the Canadian Rockies. You have a choice of a northern route to Edmonton, with a stopoff at Jasper, or a southern route to Calgary, with a stop-off at Banff and Lake Louise — both worthwhile. Get off the train at Edmonton or Calgary and fly home, for the scenery stops there.

Caribbean — It's fairly inexpensive and very accessible. Just pick an island. Or pick a ship and see several islands. The climate at sea is great year-round, but the islands themselves can get sticky in the summer.

There's no language problem — English is the native tongue on many tourist islands like Jamaica and the Bahamas, though you may have trouble with the accent. On the others, it's likely to be French.

Best deals for mature travelers are in cruises. The cruiselines have too many ships there, and so prices are dropping — in some cases, you can cruise for less than $100 a day. In addition, at least four lines that cruise the Bahamas out of southern Florida ports have posted senior-citizen discounts (see Chapter 13, Cruising). They're great for short breaks, ranging from just a day at sea to a full week or more.

Florida — The whole state, for lots of good reasons, is a mecca for mature travelers. The climate, generally, is benign, the traveling cheap and the attractions abundant. A drawback: many senior travelers complain Florida is getting too crowded. With senior travelers. And, yes, it's generally hot and muggy in the summer, though tolerable (and even lower priced).

There are lots of different Floridas, therefore lots of things to stretch out your visit. In addition to the famous things you've heard of, like Disney World, Florida is spring-training host for almost half the major-league baseball teams, and you can see exhibition games for absurdly low prices. Golf courses are abundant. And there are hundreds of miles of powder-sand, shell beaches to get lost on. There are horse racing and dog racing and jai alai to whet your betting appetite.

Florida merchants seem to love seniors. Wherever you go in Florida, you will find most hotels and motels — cheap enough as it is — offering even better rates to mature travelers. Restaurants, too. And almost every attraction. Some cities like Orlando put out senior-citizen discount books — just find a visitor's information center and ask for one.

The best way to see Florida is by driving. There are RV parks all over the place, and you should have no trouble finding a campsite even without advance reservations.

Use a central place like Orlando as a base. Spend a few days there visiting Epcot Center, Disney World, Marine World, Busch Gardens and other regional attractions. Spend a few more days driving to Miami, then on down the keys to Key West. When you return to Miami, take a day-cruise to Freeport in the Bahamas (see Chapter 13, Cruising). On the way back from Miami, cut through the Everglades on Alligator Alley (I-75) to the west coast, on up to Tampa-St. Pete, then back to Orlando. On another trip, drive north to Daytona Beach, on the coast, then up through St. Augustine (which claims to be the oldest community in the country) to Jacksonville, back down through Gainesville to the west coast, then back again to Orlando. On your way home, drive west on U.S. 98 through Panama City and Pensacola to Mobile. You will have seen some of the most interesting country in the Southeast, and probably passed near 99 percent of the retirement places in Florida.

National Parks — Motorcoach tours to places like Yellowstone, Yosemite, Zion and Grand Teton are mature travelers' favorites, tour operators tell us. And if you're driving and 62 or older, a Golden Age pass will get you free admission to the parks, as well as 50 percent off camping fees (see Chapter 11, The RV Lifestyle).

But why drive, when somebody else can do it for you? A typical motorcoach tour lasts nine days, visits three Western parks plus a few national monuments, for around $760. Motorcoaches can go almost anywhere in our national parks, and there's a minimum of walking — unless you want to walk. On some tours, you'll overnight at the most famous inns in the west — the Bright Angel Lodge at the Grand Canyon, Old Faithful Lodge in Yellowstone, Buffalo Bill's Irma Hotel in Cody and the grand Ahwanee Hotel in Yosemite.

Visiting the parks is a trip the grandkids will love. Take them along in your RV. Or check out Grandtravel's 14-day tour that ranges from Mount Rushmore to the Grand Canyon, including some horseback riding, for around $2,300.

Ozarks — There are 2 million people living in these craggy hills and deep woods in the corner where Missouri, Oklahoma

305

and Arkansas come together, almost half them retirees who came from somewhere else. And they are there for a reason: low costs, good fishing, lots of resorts (some very fancy) with good restaurants, lots of campgrounds, good live music.

And not just hillbilly music, either. With the emphasis in Nashville turning away from performing to recording, Branson, Mo., is rapidly becoming the live-country-music capital of America.

There is little flat area in the Ozarks — it's all hills and valleys. And hundreds of streams and rivers meander through. Yes, with all that water around, it gets muggy in the summer, but you tend to forget it when you're sitting in the shade fighting a big crappie on the other end of your line, walking through the deep woods or exploring an Indian cave. Here, you can teach your grandkids to fish, to water ski, to swim, to cook over a campfire. You can show them how to avoid snakes and poison ivy and how to safely row a boat. This is not an area to speed through — you have to get out of your car, follow the individual butterfly, to appreciate the Ozarks and its pace of life. If you just want to relax and play golf or tennis, the area has the resort cities of Hot Springs and Fayetteville, Ark. There are also lots of comfortable resorts around lakes like Table Rock, Bull Shoals and Tenkiller in Oklahoma. RV parks abound.

This is a driving trip. There are no cruiseships, commercial jets — not even a passenger train — in the Ozarks. Springfield, Mo., is the gateway to this part of the Ozarks. Drive to Springfield from St. Louis or Kansas City; along the way, pick up a good, detailed map of the area. Some of the finest drives are among the spiderweb of lake roads that just don't show up in an atlas.

Spain — Low-cost Spain, for Americans, is a land of great surprises for mature travelers, most of them nice ones. Because of its low cost of living and moderate climate, Spain is noted as an international retirement haven.

Spain is a big place; and mountains carve it into several different Spains.

The eastern and southern coastal areas have a mild Mediterranean climate — good for visits all year. Central Spain is arid — cold and windy in winters, hot during summers. Extreme northeastern Spain, in the Pyrenees Mountain border region, is ski country in winters. Everyone who's been anywhere in Spain warns: Beware the summer sun.

The Spanish are purposefully laid back, and go out of their way to be helpful. As one traveler said, a Spaniard would rather point you down the wrong road than admit he couldn't help you with directions.

If it's your first trip to Spain, take a tour that includes at least Seville, Córdoba, Madrid and the Costa del Sol. A nine-day tour from New York, for example, costs as little as $1,000 — including airfare. Try to see the Rioja wine region, Barcelona and San Sebastián, in the Basque country, as well, to really get a feel for the part of Spain you like. If it's summer, include Pamplona in northern Spain on your tour; the second week in July there is the San Fermin Festival — the running of the bulls. Fewer tours to these northern places, so you may have to venture there on your own.

Once you know the country, settle in somewhere, get a car and tour. One of Saga Holidays' most popular extended vacations for mature travelers is to the Costa del Sol, Spain's southern coast on the Mediterranean: 31 nights, including airfare, a London visit and some local touring, for around $1,800. And you can extend your stay for $130 a week or so. AARP has a similar package.

Renting a car to explore southern Spain is inexpensive. And be sure to spend at least a night or two in a parador — one of the old castles or monasteries the government has converted into tourist lodgings. Some run as little as $50 a night.

Texas — It's big and varied, rich in history and folklore, and not very expensive. We find the Hill Country, behind the Austin-San Antonio axis, particularly charming — unlike the parched Texas you're used to on TV's *Dallas*. It's LBJland, and they try not to let you forget it. It's remindful of the Ozarks — little lakes and rivers pop up everywhere — and there's a new vista with almost every twist of the road.

Even transient seniors fit right in with the enormous snowbird community along the Lower Rio Grande Valley, between McAllen and South Padre Island — they call the Yankees who come there for months at a time "Winter Texans," and they seem to mean it.

It's a great RV trip in the winter. Just meander all the way down I-35, through Dallas-Ft. Worth, Austin and San Antonio, then take a left at Laredo, to see the very best of Texas. That's a road that will take you all the way down the Rio Grande River to it's outlet near South Padre Island. You can day-trip into the Mexican border cities of Reynosa and Matamoros, spend a half-day seeing the warbirds of Confederate Air Force in Harlingen, and soak up some winter sunshine on the beaches of South Padre before returning home.

And don't forget to see the Alamo show in San Antonio — for Yankees, it explains a lot about why a Texan is a Texan.

Washington, D.C. — One of the world's prettiest cities and, for an American, one of its headiest. We like to sit on the steps of Mr. Lincoln's memorial at night, watch the lights of the Capitol shimmer over the Reflecting Pool, as Mr. Lincoln does, and ponder whether he approves it all. Once we spent most of a half-day at the Archives, simply watching the model of the Declaration of Independence move up and down into its nuke-proof vault. Except for the Pentagon, all the famous buildings — Capitol, White House, Library of Congress and so on — are open to visitors. Plan at least two days to give the Smithsonian a fair look. The National Gallery can take almost as long.

We like Washington for its day-trip possibilities, too. Visit Williamsburg, Baltimore, Chesapeake Bay's East Shore in a day; overnight to Philadelphia and Valley Forge, Richmond, even New York.

Best time to visit is in the spring when it's not too hot, the cherry trees are in bloom, Congress is in session and the mosquitoes aren't. You can usually watch the House or Senate from the galleries. Avoid the place in August — it's sticky then, and nobody ever seems to be in town, anyway, except tourists.

Hotels and restaurants are expensive, but there are often good weekend deals and special hotel discounts for seniors. You find these bargains in the *Washington Weekends* brochure; write Convention and Visitors Association, 1575 Eye St., N.W., Washington, DC 20005, ☎ 800/422-8644. You can also get information on deals for senior citizens at the Visitor Information Center, 1455 Pennsylvania Ave., N.W., about a block from the White House.

Washington becomes more affordable on a motorcoach tour — a typical seven-day trip that starts from New York and includes Philadelphia, Annapolis, Gettysburg and Valley Forge, costs around $700. You get only a cursory look at Washington, though — two days, not nearly enough time to see the place.

IN SUMMARY:

— There is no such thing as "a favorite place for seniors."
— But there a dozen or so places we think are special.

NOTES

CHAPTER 24

SPECIAL ADVENTURES

It's Fun to Take Trips With Your Fellow Nuts

Truly, everyone is a nut about something — golfing, fishing, biking, stamp collecting, gardening, rockhounding — and many more obscure pursuits.

Mature travelers find ways to take trips with their fellow nuts and share their special adventures. It's usually more fun to go with a group you know and share a common interest with.

ORGANIZING YOUR OWN TOUR

Recently a reader wrote our newsletter, *The Mature Traveler*: "Our round-dance club desires to take a cruise along the Mexican Riviera . . . Can you recommend a seven-day cruise departing Los Angeles or San Diego with a few interesting ports of call which would also provide a separate room for round dancing during the evening hours? There are approximately 15 couples, and we'd like to offer our caller and his wife free passage, or at least a reduced rate."

(We put her in touch with Tortuga Express of Anaheim, Calif., whose owner, Fred McLean, said he puts together dance trips like that all the time.)

If you belong to a club that has a special interest, you can organize your own group tour. Perhaps your church circle wants to visit the Holy Land, meet the Pope or hear the Mormon Tabernacle Choir. Maybe your bowling league wants a final roll-off at Bally's in Las Vegas. Maybe your investment club wants to tour the New York Stock Exchange, or watch pork bellies being traded at the Merc in Chicago.

All you have to do is contact the group-tour department of any airline, hotel or tourist agency — or a group-tour operator. El Al Israel Airlines could organize that trip to the Holy Land, for example. Bally's convention sales department might fix you up for the bowling week. Days Inn has a special department that will organize motorcoach tours for September Days members, and extra discounts on stays at Days Inns. But you'll save a lot of hassle if you put the project in the hands of a qualified travel professional, who knows all the available sources.

Your tour operator will need the same kind of information you use when planning your own trips: where you want to go, what you want to do, how much you want to spend. Your tour operator also will need to know approximately how many people you can expect to take the trip, something about your special interest and your group's level of experience. Otherwise, how can your agent plan any of those extra treats that make group travel so special?

Customarily, tour operators will give one free trip for every so many tickets sold. So if you can organize, say, 15 couples, you and your mate might go free, as the "tour leaders." But one couple we know who leads trips for their dancing club at Sun City West use the "free seat" to reduce everyone's cost by 1/16th. And once, instead, they used it for tip money aboard ship.

If your group is large enough, your travel agent can arrange special events for you — a behind-the-scenes tour of the opera, dinner with a celebrity and the like.

If you become the trip's ramrod, though, remember that you really will be the tour leader in the eyes of your friends — even if your travel agent has organized every detail. You may not want that responsibility if someone's bags get lost, if the food is terrible one night, or if your people miss the bus to the ballgame.

You may be more comfortable if someone else takes the leadership. Or if you just book an existing special-interest trip.

FINDING A SPECIAL-INTEREST TRIP

It's hard to think of a subject for which someone has not already created a special-interest trip. Many are regularly scheduled, like big-band cruises, foliage tours, gambler specials to Nevada or safaris to East Africa. Others are one-time trips, like the recent Golf Cruise With the Senior Pros that benefited the American Heart Association. And trips also can be tailor-made to suit your own interests and timing.

One of the best sources of information on special trips in your own field of interest is the *Specialty Travel Index* semiannual directory of special interest travel. You'll find the directory, in magazine format, at some libraries and at almost every travel agency. You can also send $5 (including postage) for the most current copy to Specialty Travel Index, 305 San Anselmo Ave., Ste. 217, San Anselmo, CA 94960.

A recent issue listed 6,000 or more specialty tours in 180 categories. They included antiques, archaeology, architecture, birdwatching, castles, crafts tours, camel safaris, dude ranching, computer trips, farmstays, festivals, gourmet cooking tours, golf, geology, elephant riding, llama packing, mystery tours, shopping, gem collecting, gay tours, history tours, military tours, miniatures, veterans' tours, nudist trips, whalewatching, sports tours, textile arts, wine tasting — even space travel (scheduled by Society Expeditions, departing Oct. 12, 1992 — hurry, seats are limited).

SPECIAL TRIPS THAT SENIORS TAKE

Here's a sampling of special-interest trips especially popular among mature travelers:

Learning Trips — "Learning holidays appeal to adults with an appetite for travel and a thirst for knowledge," says Henry C. Kahn, president of San Francisco's American Institute for Foreign Study. "They are the kind of people who regularly take adult courses at the local community college."

Earthwatchers (680 Mount Auburn Watertower, Box 403, Belmont, MA 02272) dig for pots beneath pueblo ruins in New Mexico, count butterflies in a Yucatan forest, measure turtles on St. Croix, photograph wildflowers in British Columbia.

Elderhostelers (80 Boylston St., Ste. 400, Boston, MA 02116) study mining methods in Nevada, theater in Indiana, stress management in Oregon, silk-weaving in India.

At an "educational vacation" week in Washington, put on for 49ers plus by Close Up Foundation (Dept. TMT, 1235 Jefferson Davis Hyway, Arlington, VA 22202), travelers have two or three seminars a day with key Washington figures, daily background briefings, a day on Capitol Hill and daily discussion groups. There's also time for touring the city's landmarks and meeting individually with your congressman or senator.

And those are only a few. A book, *The Learning Traveler: Vacation Study Abroad*, lists almost 1,000 programs offered by U.S. and foreign colleges, universities and other institutions, like Elderhostel and Earthwatch. Send $19.95 plus postage to the Institute of International Education, 341 Sutter St., Suite 510, San Francisco, CA 94104.

Adventure Travel — These appeal to mature travelers who've taken a lot of conventional trips and are looking for something new. According to Lars-Eric Lindblad, probably the dean of adventure travel, "We don't target the mature traveler, but rather the 'traveling curious' — people with a special interest, which may be nature, archaeology or even gardening."

Nevertheless, 75 percent of Lindblad Travel's clients are over 55, and on many trips the average age is closer to 65 or 70, he says, adding:

"Our clientele is not drawn from an age group so much as a state of mind."

Adventure trips can range from African safaris to polar treks to rafting the Snake River. You'll ride around in Zodiac boats and landrovers and helicopters. Adventure trips can be as soft as ballooning through Burgundy or whale watching off the Baja coast. Or as tough as backpacking in Nepal and climbing Half Dome in Yosemite.

Adventure travel isn't particularly cheap, either. Three weeks on safari in Africa can run you well over $5,000. A growing trend in adventure travel is what David Ripley, director of marketing for Sobek Expeditions based at Angels Camp, Calif., calls "super-deluxe adventure travel" — tours planned "almost exclusively for the 50-plus affluent group who like to cap a day of adventure with cocktails and clean sheets."

Along with Lindblad Travel, the leading adventure travel packagers are Abercrombie & Kent, Hemphill-Harris and

Society Expeditions. But you must get their catalogs from your travel agent. They don't book direct.

Spa Vacations — You will be pampered, petted, pushed, pinched, covered with mud, dipped in mineral water, steamed, broiled and pummeled. You'll love every minute of it. You may even return home more beautiful, or skinnier — certainly healthier. But the real object of a spa vacation is to lie back and enjoy. The problem with spa vacations, according to Jeffrey Joseph of Spa Finder, is that you can't find them. "The spa market is a whole segment that has been overlooked by agents because they are unfamiliar with how to book and sell a spa," he says. "Likewise, most spas do not market directly to agents."

So Spa Finders has put out a catalog listing more than 300 spas, most of them in the United States, along with prices, hotel accommodations and tour packages. Get it free from Spa Finder, 784 Broadway, New York, NY 10003. A more complete listing, including spas in 30 countries, several Caribbean islands and two cruiseships, is in *Spas: The International Spa Guide* by Joseph H. Bain and Eli Dror (BDIt, Inc., 1988, $12.95 in bookstores).

And, of course, there are a few spa listings in *Specialty Travel Index*.

Culture Trips — You can take in every play around London, see every important museum in Europe, hear every opera company in Italy. The Miami ballet has rehearsed and given instructions on Caribbean cruises, and Society Expeditions regularly puts scholars aboard its cruiseships to lecture passengers on topics like Eskimo history, geology and archeology.

Some museums use culture travel as fund raisers. New York's Whitney Museum of American Art sponsored a trip to view important galleries in Paris, Bordeaux, Zurich and Basel at a cost of $6,750 — that included a whopping donation to the Whitney.

Dailey-Thorp Travel, Inc., packages a wide variety of culture tours. One of the most elaborate is an opera-lovers trip to England on the QE2 with a leading singer from New York's Metropolitan Opera, with a return on the Concorde. For $9,000, you also get opera and theater tickets, a trip to Ascot for the races and a private fashion show at Fortnum & Mason. For a catalog, write Dailey-Thorpe Travel, Inc., 315 W. 57th St., Park Towers South, New York, NY 10019.

Leaf-Watching Trips — In addition to the typical foliage trip by motorcoach through New England, mounted by countless tour packagers, *Specialty Travel Index* lists leaf-watching tours of California, Colorado, Hawaii, Peru, China, Fiji and Japan.

And you're not limited to motorcoach. Several cruise companies out of New York and Boston run small ships up the New England coast and down to Washington in the autumn. And you can also take walking tours through the Vermont woods, around the Great Lakes and through Yosemite.

To shop a wide variety of foliage tours, talk with you travel agent.

Photo Trips — There are hundreds of organized photography tours to every corner of the world, some of them organized as college seminars, others just as group travel.

Typical is Photo Adventure Tours, with recent trips to Iceland, India, New Mexico, the national parks and the Caribbean. A professional photographer leads the tours and gives lessons and critiques. Book through your travel agent.

Ski Trips — Every lodge and tour packager offers ski trips in the winter, but the Over the Hill Gang (OHG) is special for mature travelers. You have to be over 50 to join.

OHG sponsors a yearly trip to the Alps just for members, and a couple of weeks each year in Colorado at reduced rates. Local chapters also have short ski trips, in addition to summer adventures like sailing, hiking, snorkeling and golfing.

An individual membership is $25 — add $15 for a spouse. Write OHG International at 13791 E. Rice Place, Aurora, CO 80015.

Retirement Trips — Before retiring to some warm place, many mature travelers like to visit several different retirement spots to see which suits them best.

The Sun City communities in Arizona and Florida (and soon in Nevada and California) have low-cost, week-long vacation packages so you can get acquainted. For information on short stays at Sun City West near Phoenix and Sun City Vistoso near Tucson, write Del E. Webb Development Co., Reservations Department, P.O. Box 1705, Sun City West, AZ 85372-1705. ☎ toll-free 800/528-2604. For trips to Sun City Center, near Bradenton, Fla., write Sun City Center Inn, P.O. Box 5698, Sun City Center, FL 33571-9989. ☎ toll-free 800/237-8200.

If you think you might to be a "Winter Texan" — one of the 200,000 snowbirds who make winter nests in the Lower Rio Grand Valley — you can take a two- or three-week drive to that area between McAllen, Texas, and South Padre Island and actually meet and play with some Winter Texans. Write the McAllen Chamber of Commerce, 10 N. Broadway, P.O. Box 790, McAllen, TX 78502 for information on retirement throughout the valley and for the free *Winter Texan Coupon Book,* full of get-acquainted deals for 49ers plus from local merchants.

Retirement Explorations runs trips for mature travelers who want to check out retirement abroad — most recently to Mexico, Portugal, Spain and Costa Rica. Write 19414 Vinyard Lane, Saratoga, CA 95070.

Rimco International and others package retirement-planning trips to Mexico, mostly the Guadalajara area including Lake Chapala, Ajijic and Tlaquepaque, popular *gringo* retirement spots. Rimco has also started an International Retirement Convention and Exposition on Mexico in Guadalajara. Write Rimco International, Inc., at Apartado Postal 1-1015, 44100 Guadalajara, Jal., Mexico, or book through your travel agent. Other Mexico trips are put on by Mexico Study Groups, P.O. Box 56982, Phoenix, AZ 85079; and Barvi Tours (Tour for Retirement in Mexico), 11658 Gateway Blvd., Los Angeles, CA 90064.

For trip planning, two good guides to retirement spots are Boyer's and Savageau's *Retirement Places Rated* (see Chapter 4, Armchair Travel) and John Howells' *Retirement Choices: For the Time of Your Life* (Gateway Books, $10.95 in bookstores).

We believe that casually visiting a place is one thing — you do it for the pleasure. But doing retirement research is something else — that's serious.

Visit your prospective retirement spot during the worst season you plan to live there. If it's Arizona or Florida, see it in the summer; if it's the Minnesota lake region, visit in the winter.

Genealogy Trips — Many make a hobby of tracing their family trees as far back as possible. And it leads to some interesting travel adventures. We talked to an American spending a week in London, mostly at the Admiralty and at Lloyd's ship registry, trying to trace a relative whose ship had gone down in a storm off Hong Kong 150 years earlier.

At the huge Mormon genealogy library in Salt Lake City, we met a man who came from Houston several times each winter with his kids. The kids would ski while the father researched his family tree. He said he'd traced one relative back to 16th-century England before he lost the trail.

You don't really have to travel to trace your own family tree. The Church of Jesus Christ of Latter-day Saints (the Mormons) maintains hundreds of centers around the country, mostly at public libraries, tied by computer into the Family History Library in Salt Lake City. But if you're into genealogical research, it's awesome to contemplate the number of records filed there. One researcher estimated there are at least two billion people on record at Salt Lake. The Mormons say most of the records contained in other genealogical libraries around the world are also at the Family History Library.

Nevertheless, there are other places in this country to visit to check out your ancestors. In Denver, Kansas City and San Francisco, the federal government has branch offices of the National Archives. In Washington, D.C., the Daughters of the American Revolution Library, near the White House, has 80,000 volumes of local histories, names and birth records dating before the Revolution. Other sources for finding your roots around Washington are the National Genealogical Society Library in Arlington and the Society of the Cincinnati Library at 2118 Massachusetts Ave. N.W.

The thing about genealogical research is that once you start, there's no stopping place. You'll find helpful librarians who direct you to other sources who direct you to other sources . . . and so on, endlessly.

Many return to Great Britain to find their roots. The Hyde Park Genealogical Library is another huge Mormon repository in London. It has records for all the British Isles. If you believe your ancestor was an important person, the College of Arms on Queen Victoria Street has a complete record of heraldic history.

An important source you can visit if your ancestors came from Europe is the Historic Emigration Office in Hamburg, Germany — more than five million emigrants from northern Europe sailed out of Hamburg from 1850 to 1914, and the office has all the ship's passenger manifests. And there are lots of other sources around the world.

Your genealogical search might lead you to a graveyard in the Ozarks, a cottage in Brittany, a tiny shrine in China, a hut in Africa — you never know where you'll need to travel, once you start. That's the joy of it.

OTHER SPECIAL TRIPS

Our list just scratches the surface of special-interest trips for mature travelers.

How could we leave out the special Bingo Bus trips from Cleveland and other Midwest cities into the Great Smokies, Royal Cruise Lines' recent Pain-Control Cruise, motorcoach trips to the Sedona, Ariz.,vortexes or the "Gone to the Dogs" Caribbean cruise for pet-lovers, on which canines were charged full fare to stay in cabins while their owners sailed free — in the same cabins, of course.

As far as we know, all these trips are chock full o'nuts. Bingo nuts, bad-back nuts, vortex nuts, dog nuts. Nuts like you and us. Everybody's a nut about something, remember? The travel insider has fun with it.

IN SUMMARY:

— It's more fun traveling with a group that shares your special interests.
— Somewhere, there's a trip planned for almost every special interest.
— Use a travel agent to help arrange your own special-interest group tour.

NOTES

CHAPTER 25

PRESERVING THE MEMORIES

Trips You Take Can Last Forever

The best thing about the journeys we've made is that each has become part of us in one way or another.

Some trips — like the one we took to Venice — yielded spectacular photos that now decorate our home. Others — like our trip to Amsterdam — resulted in a change in our lifetime breakfast pattern from ham and eggs to bread and cheese.

Still others — like our first jaunt to London — introduced us to a friend we still communicate with.

We have a quirky piece of art from Sun Valley, a golf towel from Kiawah Island, and . . . the list goes on to include a new interest acquired in one place or a piece of jewelry found in another.

THE SOUVENIRS

Perhaps you can tell from this list of things that capture our travel memories that we're not much into buying the typical souvenirs. Basically we don't much like the idea of cluttering our home with things that need to be dusted.

As a result, our collectible memories are very specific — and useful. The lady traveler likes bracelet charms that represent the places being visited. They take up almost no space, and the collection can grow at random. The gentleman traveler likes to find old maps of the country or city he's visited or to discover a local wine that he can also find and drink at home. When our favored collectibles are not available, we look for things we can use regularly.

PICTURES PERFECT

Most often, however, we rely on words and pictures of some sort to record what we've seen and done and liked.

If you're serious about taking trophy pictures — shots you can blow up, maybe even poster size, to hang on your wall — we recommend a camera a little more advanced than a Brownie box. Even expensive cameras are so automated nowadays, a beginner can work them.

We're not professional photographers — just pretty good amateurs — and so we feel we don't need a lot of extra equipment. We each carry an Olympus 35mm single-lens reflex camera — not a super-expensive model, and not a throwaway, either. One of us carries a wide-angle lens for close-quarter shots, the other a zoom telephoto lens for faraway things — and that's all. Because we have identical cameras, we can borrow each other's special lenses.

While we'd recommend a 35mm camera to everyone, we have seen travelers quite happy with Polaroids — those cameras that turn out instant color prints. For one thing, you can keep shooting a subject until you know you've got a good photo. For another, you can use the photos for trade goods: give a youngster — or even an oldster — a photo of himself, and he may trade you anything: his cap, his scarf, his ski badge, his spear . . . Or, he may pose for more photos free of charge.

Not everyone wants to be burdened with a camera and film, of course. For those people, we suggest a collection of picture postcards. Not only do they catalog where you've been in a very handsome way, the sights are all identified. Even better, postcards are easy to file and store. And if you tire of them or want to clean out the file, you can use them to write someone.

Another option is to buy professional slides. They are often available in sets of 6 to 12 at souvenir or gift shops in tourist areas. The photos are usually taken from the best vantage point for each attraction and the color is consistently good — usually better than you or we could shoot.

When we began taking our own photos, that's all we did. Shoot . . . and forget until we got home and realized our memories had often failed us when it came time to identify where or when we had taken each picture.

Now we have a system. For example, we know that when each picture or slide is developed, it will have a number on it. The number identifies the order in which the photos were taken. In other words, picture 1 was taken before picture 13. And each time we begin a new roll of film or start photographing a new locale, we take an identifying picture. We literally take a picture of the sign leading into the city or the sign outside the store or the street sign. Or do as a friend of ours does — he writes the name of the locale on a piece of paper and then takes a picture of the piece of paper before starting to photograph the scenery.

This sort of record-keeping — combined with keeping each roll of film or slides together in a box or in acetate slide-holding pages — goes a long way toward helping our memories function.

We shoot slides most often. And we've found the easiest way to keep them in order is to use what professionals call a "sleeve" — acetate pages that have pockets for each slide. We can then write identifications on tape on the outside of each pocket or on the slide mount itself. If you shoot pictures and need to store them when you get home, a box about the size of a shoebox could be ideal. Not only can you file each picture in the order it was taken, but you can use dividers to keep your trips or countries separate. A shoebox is fairly portable and takes up little space. But it should be kept in a dry area away from bright light.

If you choose to keep your pictures in albums, look for those that librarians consider "archivally safe." In other words, albums that will not accelerate the aging or deterioration process. For example, albums that have adhesive on their pages incorporate chemicals that will make your pictures fade or bleed.

THE ELECTRONIC ERA

Everywhere we go we see our fellow travelers carrying tape recorders, movie cameras and video camcorders. That's far more lugging than we want to do when we're traveling. But we can understand the desire to capture it "like it is."

323

Before buying this kind of equipment, research it carefully. Electronic gear seems to go out of date even before it makes it to the store shelf. You may want to buy the equipment from a discounter, but do your shopping at a full-service store where you touch and feel the device, work the levers and talk to an expert.

Also consider renting the equipment at your location. Many areas that host visitors offer rental camcorders so you don't have to pack and carry them.

But before you use this kind of gear, be sure it is allowed. Many attractions attempting to preserve rare collections or to cope with copyright laws prohibit the use of recorders, as well as flash cameras.

Of the electronic gear available, we use the hand-held mini tape recorders most often. Its like taking notes with your voice, and the recorder is small enough to fit into a purse or pocket. We generally resort to the tape recorder when it's too dark to see to write, or if it's too cold to hold a pencil.

MEMORIES ARE MADE OF THIS

The best way we keep the memories of our travels clear is to write them down when they are fresh. Each of us uses a different style, but the results are the same: a diary we can read years later that helps us call to mind details that may be on the verge of slipping away.

The gentleman traveler uses a pocket-size looseleaf notebook to jot down his thoughts as he goes. Often, his photo identifications wind up in this same notebook, side by side with the notes he's made about the people we've met or the unusual things we've seen.

The lady traveler prefers the small, bound notebooks filled with crisp, white, empty pages. With this kind of notebook, each trip has its own diary of the good, bad and indifferent. The notebooks are not expensive, but they do make a colorful section on a home bookshelf. They're filled with moods and reactions to the new things encountered in new places — sometimes even entire menus — whatever describes the events that made the trip memorable.

KEEPING IT SIMPLE

Whatever your choice for recording your trip — or for the devices you use to record your memories — keep it simple. Otherwise you're likely to spend most of your powers of concentration dealing with the equipment, not with the travel experience.

If there's one message we want you to keep from this book it is this:

Keep it simple.

Don't burden yourself with the unfamiliar or untried — shoes, luggage, clothes, equipment.

The experiments and adventures should be in the journey, itself.

ABOUT *THE MATURE TRAVELER* NEWSLETTER
Save $2.50 on the Subscription Price

Pinning down great discounts and entertaining trips for mature travelers is like shooting at a moving target — they come and go too frequently for any book to describe completely. Reading a good monthly newsletter is the only way to keep abreast of the latest good news — discounts, trips, great places and good advice — for mature travelers. And we believe our own newsletter, *The Mature Traveler* is the best one you'll find anywhere.

In appreciation for purchasing our book, *Get Up and Go* **we'll give you $2.50 off your first-year's subscription to** *The Mature Traveler***. Just use this coupon.**

....

_____YES! I want to subscribe to **The Mature Traveler**. I understand that if I use this coupon as a purchaser of *Get Up And Go* I will get $2.50 off the regular $21.97 subscription price.

_____My check for $19.47 for one year is enclosed, OR

Charge my _____ Visa _____Mastercard.

Card No._____Expires_____

SIGNATURE_____

NAME_____

ADDRESS_____

CITY_____ STATE_____ ZIP_____

Mail to: The Mature Traveler, P.O. Box 50820, Reno, NV 89513.

GATEWAY BOOKS
31 Grand View Avenue
San Francisco, CA 94114

Our books for mature travelers and mature stay-at-homes are available in most bookstores. However, if you have any difficulty finding them, we will be happy to ship them to you directly.

Mail us this coupon with your check or money order and they'll be in the mail to you within days.

Get Up and Go:	$10.95	_____
A Guide for the Mature Traveler		
Choose Mexico:	9.95	_____
Retire on $400 a Month		
Choose Latin America	9.95	_____
A Guide to Seasonal and Retirement Living		
Retirement Choices:	10.95	_____
For the Time of Your Life		
To Love Again:	7.95	_____
Intimate Relationships After 60		
Subtotal::		_____

Add $1.50 for postage and handling for the first book, $ .50 for each additional one. (California residents add 6% sales tax.)   _____

Total Enclosed.. $_____

NAME_____

ADDRESS_____

CITY_____STATE_____ZIP_____

Mail to: Gateway Books, 31 Grand View Avenue San Francisco, CA 94114